HEALING
A LIFE WITH CHRONIC ILLNESS

"This is a sensitive and moving journey into the despair and hope of the frightening challenges facing a person with a misunderstood, debilitating disease, interstitial cystitis. The writer is an unusually perceptive individual who links the medical to the social aspects of illness. Health professionals stand to gain from the great insights of this book."
—T. C. Theoharides, Ph.D., M.D.,
Professor of Pharmacology, Internal Medicine, and Biochemistry;
Associate Professor of Psychiatry at the Tufts University School of Medicine,
New England Medical Center

"Marguerite Bouvard draws upon a wealth of talent and experience as an author to describe her own journey with a chronic debilitating condition. By going beyond coping to a higher level of personal healing, this inspiring book offers important insights to all who suffer with chronic illness, their family and friends, and also for healthcare workers."
—Paul Church, M.D., Urology Department, Faulker Hospital

"Interstitial Cystitis is a devastating chronic illness that exists with a number of other auto-immune diseases. This compelling story of one woman's arduous journey shows how the mind-body connection can provide healing and help rebuild a rewarding life. I highly recommend it."
—Kristine Whitmore, M.D.,
Professor of Urology and OB/GYN, Drexel University

"Marguerite Bouvard shows us how living with chronic illness can be a gateway into the soul. Her story touches our hearts and creates a place inside ourselves for true healing to begin."
—Rev. Dr. Samuel Oliver, *What the Dying Teach Us: Lessons on Living*

HEALING

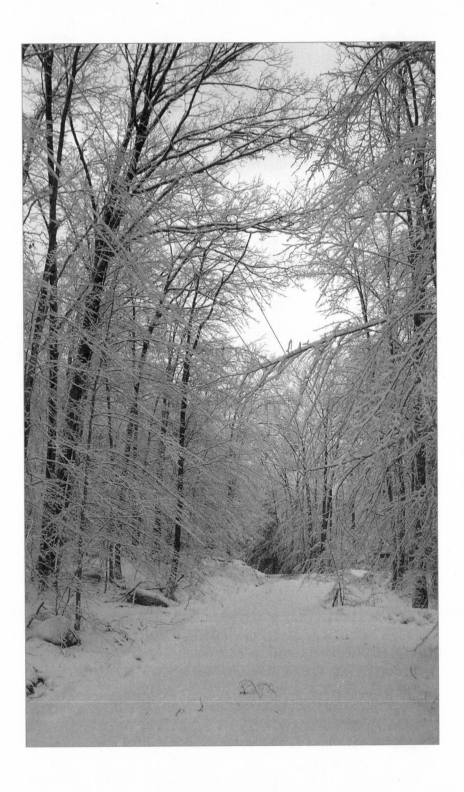

HEALING

A LIFE WITH
CHRONIC ILLNESS

Marguerite Guzmán Bouvard

University Press of New England
Hanover and London

Published by University Press of New England,
One Court Street, Lebanon, NH 03766
www.upne.com
© 2007 by Marguerite Guzmán Bouvard
Printed in the United States of America
5 4 3 2 1

Text design and photograph on page ii by Joyce Weston.

Library of Congress Cataloging-in-Publication Data
Bouvard, Marguerite Guzman, 1937–
  Healing : rebuilding a life with chronic illness / Marguerite Guzman Bouvard.
    p. cm.
ISBN-13: 978–1–58465–623–4 (pbk. : alk. paper)
ISBN-10: 1–58465–623–9 (pbk. : alk. paper)
  1. Bouvard, Marguerite Guzman, 1937—Health.   2. Interstitial cystitis—Patients—Biography.   I. Title.
RC921.C9B68 2007
362.196'6230092—dc22
[B]   2006101272

 University Press of New England is a member of the Green Press Initiative. The paper used in this book meets their minimum requirement for recycled paper

To my husband

꙰꙰꙰

CONTENTS

ACKNOWLEDGMENTS

My thanks to the friends who read this manuscript and encouraged me along the way, most especially Barbara Greenberg, Helen Fremont, Mariève Rugo, and to Ethel Smith.

My gratitude to Jessica Lott, editor extraordinaire, who helped me through repeated revisions of the manuscript.

I also wish to acknowledge the physicians who have accompanied me with such understanding, most particularly Isaac Schiff, M.D., director of the Vincent Memorial Center for Obstetrics and Gynecology at the Massachusetts General Hospital, Lisa Cautillo, P.A., and Kristene Whitmore, M.D.

My thanks to Shulamit Reinharz, director of the Women's Studies Research Center at Brandeis University, for providing an environment for research that is as inclusive as it is multidisciplinary and where new insights and projects are always welcomed.

The Virginia Center for the Creative Arts has been a haven for me throughout my illness, and I wish to thank the director, Suny Monk, and especially Sheila Gulley Pleasants for her heroic efforts to make my stays both possible and comfortable.

I also wish to thank the friends who understand my physical limits with such sensitivity: Marilyn Ewer, who came up with a project when I was first diagnosed; Ana Velilla, Judy Keefe, Sheila Carchidi, and Heidi Shyu, who are always with me in spirit when I am unable to be with them and who have given me so much support.

My warmest appreciation to my husband, devoted companion, whose unstinting kindness and understanding have helped me through so many difficult times.

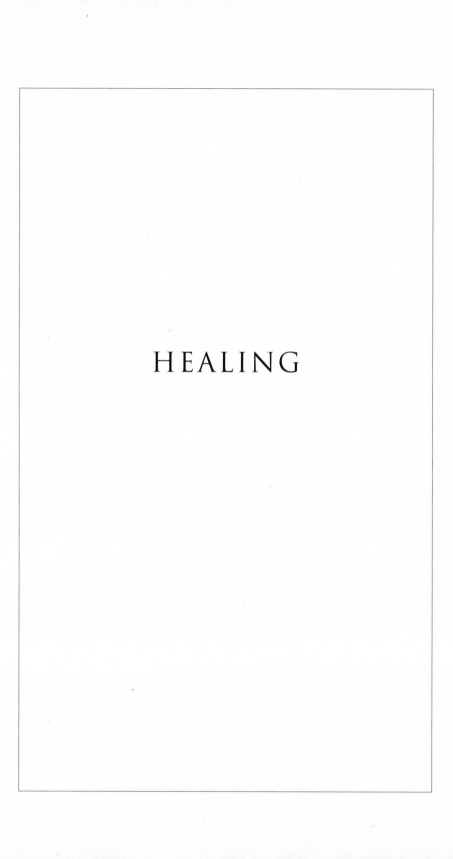

HEALING

1

A JOURNEY OF TRUE HEALING

O N E   D A Y after I had been ill for some years, I was walking down Boylston Street in Boston and saw a man stretched out sleeping in an alleyway. That vision stayed with me while I ran my errands, and I returned by the same route so that I could stop. I leaned over him and woke him up so we could talk and I could give him some money for breakfast and lunch. He was not drunk, was not a bum, as many passersby might have assumed, but one of the many homeless working poor. Startled at first, he then looked at me with a dawning acceptance and pleasure that was mutual, for we were able to recognize our travels in each other. In the time before my illness I would have regarded such a gesture as futile, would have complained about the lack of low-cost housing and of social safety nets, and would have deplored public indifference to the plight of so many. I hope a new generation is working toward change as I do on a very small scale. But my illness helped me to understand how one person contains the world, how even the wounded carry flight within. It was just one episode in a journey of learning to see the world around me in new ways.

This book is about rebuilding a life seemingly shattered by chronic illness. I found that, in so doing, I was actually deeply involved in the grieving process with its phases of denial, disorganization, and acceptance. The chaos of emotions that shook me when I least expected them was part of the hard work of grief. However, in recovering from a loss, these phases do not follow each other sequentially, nor are they self-contained. I found that while I was in the deepest denial, pretending I was well and deciding to travel to Argentina in order to write a book, that trip was also a learning experience that would help me learn how to heal myself. The Mothers of the Plaza de Mayo in Argentina would never find their children who had been killed in concentration camps, so they expressed their grief by displaying a political rage in their marches that propelled them toward a new and fulfilling life. From them I learned about the uses of anger and self-discovery in recovering from a horrendous blow. For me as well, the healing process entailed staying involved in social activism as well as learning to live mindfully and to become thankful for what I had.

The grief I felt over the loss of my health, and consequently my career and my former ease, also involved facing a crisis of meaning. In the early years I wondered what I had done to deserve this. Again, while I was questioning the injustice of such a blow and repeatedly asking myself why this was happening to me, I spent time facing an even more troubling world of injustice—the loss of the Argentine Mothers' children and a government's effort to silence them. After I returned home and started to work on my book, I found myself revising my values, questioning my views of success and even my perspective on the world. Rather than turning away from religion, my bewilderment led me on a spiritual quest that for me represented an awakening.

In the early years of my illness, writing books about human rights, which involved many interviews with activists, was a way of keeping my passions alive. When I no longer had the stamina to travel or even have a schedule, I expanded and revised my activism in ways I could physically accommodate. That was and continues to be my most effective medicine— along with learning to live in the present, in all its richness. I found that I needed to honor my interests in order to live hopefully and well. For me, living hopefully does not mean waiting for a cure, but maintaining a sense of wonder and possibility. Like so many of us who are ill, I found that my physical condition did not define me even though it transformed my lifestyle and perspectives in many ways.

At the onset of interstitial cystitis, a little-understood illness, I felt disoriented, as if I were floundering. It seemed as if I were back at school, trying to learn important subjects for survival without a teacher, or traveling in a new country without a map. In retrospect, while I was seemingly moving backward, I was actually taking leaps into the future. As I coped with the physical problems of my condition, I was simultaneously taking the risk of redefining myself, a risk I might never have taken if had remained healthy and continued rushing through my days without the opportunity for prolonged inner reflection. Nothing is more difficult than change, especially if one is content with one's circumstances. But I discovered that although it is painful, change is often a source of significant growth in all aspects of our lives.

An important part of dealing with my condition was the issue of relations with the medical profession as well as with my healthy friends and colleagues. Because I had used my office hours to help my students with their emotional issues when I was a professor, I foolishly expected a degree of understanding from the physicians I first encountered. Instead, I entered the world of distancing medical terminology and technology, feeling myself reduced to an obstreperous organ whose relationship to the rest of my body was ignored. I found myself wishing that a physician would actually make eye contact with me and acknowledge me as more than my illness. I wished that we could have a dialogue, however brief.

Rebuilding my life meant reclaiming language so I could learn to speak about the entire experience of illness, especially to members of my family and to a few close friends. Oddly, I found myself becoming their teacher. I taught them simple phrases that could help me feel accompanied, assuring them that these were all I needed, that they didn't have to feel obliged to "fix" my situation. I also learned how to be more assertive with physicians, writing out questions before a consultation and trying to achieve a greater balance in our conversations.

Learning a new language to convey the reality of my situation opened up a whole new area of working toward human rights as well as reorienting my life as a writer. I began speaking with the ill and dying in order to break down their isolation, writing articles, poems, and prayers about living with illness and physical frailty. A woman who read my book of poems, *The Body's Burning Fields*, wrote to me, "Your poetry spoke directly to me and gave me hope, knowing I am not alone. So few understand what long-term pain and suffering does." Living with illness enlarged my outlook as I came to experience a profound connection with the suffering and dispossessed around the world. It proved to be an everyday act of inclusion.

Thus, for me, healing means not only learning to take charge of my physical care but, just as important, taking charge of my own life. It means learning to live intensely and with awareness, the opposite of what so many people perceive as the truncated lifestyles of the ailing. Chronically ill people do not define their days as consisting of trips to the doctor, resting, and taking their medication. These are just strands in my routine. I have a number of friends with chronic conditions, and they are all immersed in significant work even though they tire easily. My main focus is on my writing, on reflecting and working toward a more just world. I live in the present, taking each moment as it comes, to be savored and explored for what it may hold. Although I have frequent and difficult times of pain and sleeplessness, I know that they will pass. The tapestry of life is vast, complex, and shines with its own particular beauty.

I learned too just how much I could expand my inner life. What I eventually lost in being unable to attend the events and conferences that once nourished me was compensated by the discovery of how vast the space of reflection can become. I enrich my days by tapping into my own resources, by paying attention to my surroundings, whether the changing light on the maple trees seen through my window or the faces of people in a physician's waiting room, studying the world as if I were seeing it for the first time. I also focus on the small pleasures in life such as listening to music, taking up a small project such as sewing, or returning to interests I didn't have time for in my very busy professional life. I don't believe that there is a hierarchy of interests, that some are more valuable than others. Some people may be entranced by reading Burpee seed catalogues as they dream of planting in spring even if they are unable to do so. I returned to my collection of art books that had been gathering dust in the back of my bulging bookcase and to designing and making quilts.

Most important, I found that true healing involved reconnecting what society seems to want to sever—the mind/body/heart. Since I was so often treated as merely a body-object by some physicians while I was subjected to the hurricane of emotions that attend illness, I learned to pay attention to those feelings, to respect them and work with them and move on rather than pushing them underground. Facing times of discouragement head-on helped me traverse the zigzagging of the spirit with renewed strength.

While the world around me may associate physical vulnerability with weakness, I consider myself strong and believe that my strength is made of acceptance, adaptability, and a resilient and open spirit. That is what it means to make oneself whole. Daily meditation has also helped me toward that goal and has influenced the changes in my perspective. Most people don't think of a chronically ill person as having integrated the many attributes of a human being. They see me as lesser. But in reweaving the many layers of my being, I have come to honor myself as well as my connection with all of humanity.

Although the details of my journey are unique, the underlying issues of true healing are universal. They affect us all at some periods in our lives. I believe that many people could profit from this story: caregivers, friends of the ill, and people who are subject to the vagaries of the economy and the changes in our social values. Even those who seem to sail through life with easy circumstances could find much that is useful. We could all learn that each one of us is capable of living well with sometimes daunting conditions. And that is an important lesson.

2

CROSSING THE BORDER

In May of 1987, my semester as a professor of political science at a small women's college was almost finished. With a sigh of relief I drove to Kennebunkport, Maine, as soon as I had graded all my exams and papers, stashing away mountains of course notes and packing up my computer and books so I could return to the poetry I loved writing. My daughter had just graduated from college and was off for a year at the London Academy of Music and Dramatic Arts. My son was working in California, and my husband was absorbed in his very demanding job. I felt weightless as I started the hour-and-a-half drive to Maine.

Mornings, I walked along Goose Rocks Beach as soon as I woke up. No pressing schedule, where each hour was accounted for and where I needed to rush from one task to another. No syllabi to prepare, students to worry over, or lists of things to do. The college where I worked demanded much of its professors, not so much in the classroom I loved as in endless committee meetings and the production of reports that would never be read. Thus it was a relief to be alone with the tides, the terns nesting at the far corner of the beach, and the estuarial river flexing its long tendons. I felt the crush of my hectic life melt away, gazing at the ocean until it seemed as if its blue doors were opening and there was no time at all.

The cabin I rented was rudimentary, rather like an enlarged toolshed, with a bedroom and a combination living room–kitchenette where I parked my computer on a rickety table. But it faced a salt marsh where I watched herons regally picking their way among the grasses. Nights, I listened to a local classical music station or played my Italian tapes to hold on to my first language, which I have so little opportunity to speak. I read and worked on a quilt, feeling utterly contented and complete.

Then suddenly one night I was seized with an urgency to urinate that made me get up repeatedly. That need was so acute it was not something I could sleep through or ignore. It happened the following night and then the night after, but I continued to revel in my morning and late afternoon walks because I was so energetic that interrupted nights didn't seem to bother me.

I had never paid much attention to my body. I wasn't athletic, although I loved walking, hiking, and bicycling (and this was before the fitness craze). Since I had always enjoyed good health, I took my physical ease for granted and felt secure in the belief it would always support my many pursuits, including volunteering and political activism in addition to my career. Thus when my husband came to visit at the end of my stay I didn't mention my nightly sprints through the bitter cold cabin: they didn't seem important as I was returning home with new poems.

But May became June and I was still getting up at night, often enough to make me think of contacting a doctor. I called my general practitioner, and she suggested I see the urologist she recommended. At the end of June I found myself face to face with a cheerful young specialist. When I recounted my symptoms, he told me "You just have a bladder infection," prescribing an antibiotic. I insisted that I had never had such an infection in my life and I was certain I didn't have one now because I knew that bladder infections were painful, a symptom I wasn't experiencing. He ignored my comment.

After taking the antibiotic for ten days without any change in my symptoms, I telephoned the doctor and we had a fruitless exchange. I was beginning to feel a nagging frustration, an undercurrent of fear. I called my gynecologist, who referred me to another urologist whom I visited at the end of August.

I was both trusting and ill prepared to deal with doctors. When I recounted my symptoms to the gruff person sitting across the table, he replied, "Get undressed and step inside the examining room." He didn't prepare me for what was to come, inserting a catheter in my bladder and pumping it up with water to see how much it was able to hold, an incredibly painful procedure that I later discovered is generally performed in a hospital under anesthesia.

"There's nothing wrong with you," he insisted. "Probably your uterus is pressing against your bladder. I would have it removed." I stumbled out the door in blinding pain, sensing that he had not diagnosed me properly, that it was not an unusual male reaction for someone of his generation to suggest I have my female organs removed. As soon as I came home, I lay down to recover. Then I called my gynecologist to tell her about the visit, and she was horrified.

I felt disoriented and bewildered by my symptoms and the lack of diagnosis. Because I didn't know what to do or where to turn, I took solitary walks around Lake Waban, bordering Wellesley College, to reflect on my situation. I mulled over my exchanges with the doctors I had consulted, hearing myself say again and again, "I have never been seriously ill before." If the doctors didn't know what was wrong with me, how was I supposed to know? I was frightened and confused, swinging between imagining the worst and believing my problems were a passing episode. Just as I had difficulty communicating with doctors, I was also unable to describe these new experiences to my family and colleagues. I kept returning to that lake, where light falling through the leaves reminded me of wavering stained glass. I gazed at eddies on the water as if they held an answer to my dilemma.

Gradually, my sense of taste changed significantly. The grapefruit I usually had for breakfast seemed unbearably sour, and the tomato sauces I liked to concoct also stung my taste buds. Then I began to experience a burning in my lower abdomen. That, too, I wondered at but ignored as I worked in my study, preparing my courses for the fall semester.

By now I was leading three demanding lives: my crowded teaching schedule, my project for a book on women and human rights, and the puzzling life of a body seemingly out of control. I was foolish enough to believe that somehow I could keep these strands from interfering with each other as I doggedly gave lectures that fall, arranging for guest speakers on human rights to address my classes and planning for my book while getting up to urinate sometimes as many as seven times at night and ignoring the discomfort in my lower abdomen. As far as I was concerned, that was an undertone. I have since learned from other people who were diagnosed with serious illnesses that it takes a very long period to accept the reality of a new and frightening condition.

In late October, I was sitting in our dining room with Martha, a poet friend. We were critiquing each other's poems when she suddenly told me she had received a sabbatical and was planning a trip to the Galapagos Islands. I was caught up in her enthusiasm, remembering the slide shows of those beautiful islands I once saw many years ago. "I'll come with you if you go in January between semesters," I recklessly blurted out, for I was still carrying on my life as if nothing had changed. Initially this was not a catastrophic illness that felled me like a stroke or cancer and that required known treatments. It was like the slow and gradual invasion of an army, so I was able to remain in denial.

Martha found a tour that combined airfare, hotel, and a week on a small boat. I was approaching my fiftieth birthday, and I wanted to spend it in a daring way. Part of me is a Walter Mitty, for I am skinny and uncoordinated. Throughout my school years, my gym teachers would throw up their hands in frustration at my clumsiness. Yet I have always dreamed of trekking through Nepal or climbing Mont Blanc. When I was a child, I hungrily read about the deep-sea dives of William Beebe in his bathysphere that just happened to be named *Trieste*, the city of my birth. I journeyed vicariously to Tibet with William O. Douglas and Alexandra David-Neel and to Nepal with the zoologist George Schaller, imagining myself wading knee deep through the snow for hours on end and then retiring to a soaked sleeping bag to take notes, drinking tea with rancid yak butter. Now, as I planned my Galapagos adventure, I was overwhelmed at the thought that I could actually make such a journey myself.

In no time at all, my efficient friend Martha finalized the arrangements for our travel. Yet throughout the fall I kept having misgivings about whether I could handle such a journey. There were times I wanted to postpone it because I was fatigued, too many times when I called Martha about my indecision. We were both on a tight budget, and when I told her I wanted a single room in the hotel in Quito she was justifiably concerned. I was unable to coherently explain my need for privacy and rest.

My husband finally persuaded me to take that leap. "It's a chance in a lifetime," he said. "Go ahead." Martha and I took off in the midst of a heavy snowstorm, she sporting a camera and I carrying a pair of binoculars my husband had given me as well as a bag of very useful gadgets my well-organized daughter had thoughtfully provided.

It was worth a canceled flight, an all-night delay, and the discomfort when our small plane finally landed on the Galapagos and we boarded the little boat that was to be our home for a week. Our very first morning, we clambered into a small motorboat to visit seemingly deserted Baltra Island. When I saw a family of seals lazily sunning themselves on the sand, I became so excited I forgot to watch my steps along the slippery rocks and tumbled down in a heap, denting the binoculars.

Luckily we were on a schedule that I was able to tolerate. Since interrupted sleep was my main problem at the time, I still had enough energy to sustain me during our morning expeditions. Because of the intense heat, Martha and I napped afternoons. Evenings after dinner, we read Darwin along with the other six passengers in the one common room, which had a collection of books and where the meals were served. Then we all retired early.

We did punctuate our routine with occasional celebrations. On my birthday, one of the people on our tour took a photo of Martha and me on top of a volcanic cone, arm in arm with our sun hats and our long-sleeved shirts, looking like two Englishwomen on a nineteenth-century safari, and that night the cook prepared a birthday cake and served a special wine.

But for me, the high point of our excursions was walking through a nesting site of blue-footed boobies, a bird endemic to the islands. I was utterly fascinated by the chicks vibrating their feathers to cool themselves from a punishing sun and by the pale strands of grasses, their subdued colors also an adaptation to the merciless climate. There was a transparency about the awful struggle for survival and also a triumph. At the time, responding to harsh conditions was the province of zoology and not a personal quest, although I would come to view this experience as part of learning a new language.

Martha and I spent our last days in Quito apart because I needed to rest after our journey. I spent my mornings strolling through the city, observing the crowds of youngsters in the parks and streets, for the majority of the population is under fifteen. Afternoons, I rested in my hotel room writing in the journal my daughter had given me before I left.

In retrospect, I am glad I overcame my fears and actually took that trip with Martha because it would be a time I could look back on with great pleasure. I had dreamed of doing something spectacular to celebrate my fiftieth birthday, climbing a mountain for example. Taking that small boat around the islands turned out to be my mountain—and the last time I could take such a demanding excursion.

I returned to teaching at the end of January brimming with projects. I discovered that the students in my International Relations class, who generally seemed apathetic about what was happening abroad, became interested and alive when I brought in as guest speakers women who were fighting for human rights against great odds. I invited women dissidents such as Lu Hsiu-lien, who had spent ten years in prison in Taiwan for trying to promote democratic elections. She brought a pair of slippers she

had embroidered with FREEDOM while in jail, a word her Taiwanese jail-
ers couldn't read. After class my students crowded around her, wanting
to be near the woman who had not only fought for democracy but also
founded a women's movement in a male-dominated culture. Watching my
students become excited and involved, I wanted to reach more people,
to help others outside the college also discover through such role models
that we are not powerless in this world.

I decided to write a book featuring women who had worked on behalf
of human rights, for they were still overshadowed by their male counter-
parts. I was motivated not only by my years of political activism and my
wish to inspire my students but also by my own history. I had attended
graduate school before the women's movement and was one of the first
women to graduate with a Ph.D. in political science at the then male bas-
tion of Harvard University. It was a triumph but also a very difficult experience as my professors and fellow students either tried to render me
invisible or made annoying sexual overtures. My anger at this treatment
helped awaken me to the fact that my case was not an isolated one and
that there were larger issues at stake for women, which would lead me to
write about women's rights.

My passion for this project overshadowed my changing physical condition. I even applied for a grant from my college to travel to Argentina
in order to write about the Mothers of the Plaza de Mayo. When I first
saw their photo in a *New York Times* article, a group of somber women
wearing identical white scarves and demonstrating in the plaza before the
presidential palace on behalf of their "disappeared" children, I became
obsessed with wanting to hear and research their story firsthand, for defy-
ing the government at the time meant either death or imprisonment. I
wanted to include a chapter on these women whose children had been
killed in clandestine concentration camps during the years of a brutal
military junta between 1976 and 1984 and to bring their message of empowerment to my students. I felt the Mothers' defiance and their thirst for
justice in my very bones.

Meanwhile a year passed before I had the courage to consult another
urologist. He was a kindly man and listened carefully while I recounted
my symptoms. "You probably have interstitial cystitis," he said. "I don't
want to test you for it, because it is a painful procedure and because I
am almost certain you have it." Then he said, "There's not much I can
do for you." He prescribed some Ditropan, which helps control urinary
frequency, and suggested that I adjust the dosage to suit my needs. He

also gave me the address of a support group for people who suffer from this illness.

I searched for articles on interstitial cystitis and discovered that it is an inflammation and deterioration of the bladder lining. At the time, I didn't understand that it is a chronic illness that affects women in particular—and that, because of this, I had found myself hearing the same derogatory phrases from physicians that I had heard earlier from my professors as a graduate student. And so I had spent two years listening to doctors suggest that I was simply being "emotional" before I found a urologist who took me seriously. It would take many more years for a physician to acknowledge the crushing fatigue I was living with and to identify the immune disorder that sometimes accompanies interstitial cystitis (IC) as it progresses.

IC is one of a number of autoimmune disorders such as chronic fatigue syndrome (CFS) that affect mainly women. It is poorly understood. Recently epidemiological studies have confirmed my own experience with the onset of this condition. They reveal that it takes on average five to seven years to get diagnosed and sometimes ever longer. They also confirm that because physicians are often not familiar with IC, women are frequently told that their symptoms are "all in their head" or caused by stress, thereby invalidating the pain and compounding an already devastating condition. It wasn't until 1990, three years after the onset of my symptoms, that the lack of medical research into female-specific disorders was recognized and that the National Institutes of Health opened the Office of Research on Women's Health. It took another ten years of research for physicians to realize that IC is not only about an organ but also has nerve-related links to its cause and development, affecting the whole body. Today, research has demonstrated that IC is frequently associated with other chronic conditions such as fibromyalgia/chronic fatigue syndrome, pain in the vulvar region known as vulvodynia, allergic reactions, and gastrointestinal problems. Eventually I would develop fibromyalgia and vulvodynia as well as allergic reactions, discovering that dealing with several chronic illnesses at once can be overwhelming.

But at the time, my most important recourse was to get in touch with a young woman from the support group, Laurie Brown, whom I never met in person but who became a telephone friend during this very difficult year. She called me frequently to see how I was doing and helped diminish my sense of isolation. We compared symptoms, and she gave me useful suggestions on how to deal with the burning in my abdomen by sending me a copy of a diet that was easing her own discomfort.

I found that cutting out a number of foods such as citrus, coffee, tea, chocolate, alcohol, tomatoes, processed cheese, and any kind of spices including onions and garlic proved very helpful. Unfortunately the list was a very long one, as I discovered that many sweets contained cinnamon and breads included a variety of spices. My husband suggested I keep a journal of my reactions until I found a diet that suited me. It resulted in a very bland and limited fare, an apple or pear for lunch (the only fruit I could eat without pain) plus some sweetened but unflavored yogurt, or a protein shake along with crackers for lunch. Dinner became unseasoned meat or chicken, salad without dressing, and a starch or steamed vegetables. This diet eased my daytime pain considerably but made it very difficult to eat in a restaurant or to visit friends for dinner without long and apologetic explanations. I remember trying to explain my restrictions to a nonplussed waitress. She just stared at me until I quipped, "Oh, just bring me an empty plate!"

I have since learned to carry apples and hard-boiled eggs when I travel by air and on the rare occasions I attend large gatherings that include a buffet or light meal. I also read labels with the intensity of a person consulting an encyclopedia whenever my husband and I grocery-shop. He is good-natured enough to often "taste" food for me when we are out, making certain there is nothing acidic or spicy included—and reminding me that tasting for poison was an important role for retainers under the French kings.

Laurie also gave me a list of doctors treating interstitial cystitis, with an evaluation of each one corroborated by other women who suffered from IC, almost like the underground guide to professors that students circulate among themselves at most colleges. She suggested I consult a specialist in IC who was in the forefront of research on the illness and whom she had seen.

Following Laurie's advice, I made an appointment with this physician. It was by now two years since my problems had begun, and I was still juggling work, research, and difficult nights. The physician advised me to let him do a biopsy within my bladder wall, the proven way of diagnosing the disease at the time. I entered the New England Medical Center in July 1989 with trepidation, electing to stay awake during the procedure in order to learn something.

During the biopsy, the doctor excitedly addressed his students: "Notice the accumulation of mast cells!" I wondered what mast cells were and what role they played in my condition. I didn't ask for information, foolishly believing it would be forthcoming. This was my introduction to the medical profession, where patients are supposed to be passive and compliant.

Later that afternoon the doctor confirmed that I did indeed have interstitial cystitis. He was beaming as he entered my room with his students in tow. The pain in my bladder made me feel as if I were constantly pissing broken glass, and this pain would continue for several days. He bustled off to complete his rounds, and I was left with a sense of desolation. "You're handling it very well," he commented as he swished out the door. I had been reduced to an organ that happened to be attached to an anonymous someone.

At my follow-up visit, the doctor suggested I try monthly treatments of an anti-inflammatory, DMSO. I began the DMSO treatments some months later, but they had little effect on my symptoms. The urologist then prescribed Doxepin, an antidepressant commonly used by people suffering from IC to dull the pain and help them sleep at night. It made me feel intensely nauseated. I scheduled a follow-up visit, during which he listened to my accounts of pain and sleeplessness, nodding and commenting, "These are typical of interstitial cystitis." He offered me no further help. At the time I didn't realize how puzzling IC was to many urologists because it was so newly discovered and because it had no identifiable causes.

My visits to other urologists were equally unrewarding. One of them even suggested that I have my bladder removed and a prosthesis installed. I was in tears from exhaustion while he beamed with excitement. "You'll feel so much better if you have this procedure," he predicted. "You'll even be able to have a glass of wine with your husband." I read up on the subject and discovered that there can be multiple side effects from such a drastic step, including bacterial infections. This solution is used on only 2 percent of IC sufferers and then as a last resort. Until I gathered my medical records for the insurance company the following year, I didn't know that, in addition to a chronic inflammation and deterioration of the lining, I also had a lesion in my bladder wall.

Slowly I discovered that I was supposed to be in charge, but I still didn't know where to turn next or how to proceed. I decided to stay away from specialists altogether for a time, continuing my life of teaching and planning a trip to Argentina in August to be with the Mothers of the Plaza de Mayo. I was hovering between two worlds: that of the healthy (for, despite my problems, I still considered myself to be so) and the as yet unfathomable world of people with chronic illnesses. I didn't realize that this was the beginning of learning a new culture or that I would have to create a language that would reflect my reality. Nor was I aware of one of the sources of my deep discomfort: that to become ill in this society means having the body, spirit, and mind severed. How could I speak to the people around me about my fear and anxiety, how could I speak to the self that was changing, when I was unable to find the words and had no frame of reference?

I wrote in my journal: *The image that comes to mind when I think of this juncture in my life is one of beginning a new book. It's not as people imagine, just stepping into a stream of connections where meaning unfolds like notes in a prelude. It's a condition of disorientation and chaos. I begin a sentence that barely approaches what I am trying to name. I cannot see shapes, totality or even steps in a process. But this is what beginning is and I know of no other way to find meaning.*

3

ARGENTINA

WHEN MY cousin had a biopsy in her breast that revealed a cancerous tumor, she hopped on her bicycle and went for a long ride in the countryside. It was a way of dealing with her shock and preparing herself for what lay ahead. But the diagnosis I received didn't provide me with an understanding that IC was a chronic illness, or that it could worsen. Thus, instead of taking a bicycle ride, I decided to take a plane to Buenos Aires. Buoyed by the small travel research grant I had received to fly to Argentina, I arranged a trip to visit the Mothers of the Plaza de Mayo in Buenos Aires.

Little did I suspect that traveling to the unknown would be so similar to the uncharted passage through my illness. I would discover important lessons about living with a chronic condition, how to tap into the torrent of emotions that I was experiencing and not only express them but transform them into powerful statements. I would learn from the Mothers how to overcome fear and feel empowered. In effect, I was going to a school for some important life lessons.

On August 10, 1989, I boarded Varig Airlines for my flight to São Paulo, Brazil, where I would then make a connection to Buenos Aires. That made the flight even longer, but it also made it affordable. I breathed a sigh of relief when dinner arrived and I actually was served a meal I could eat. But I felt embarrassed at trekking back and forth to the bathroom so often as if everyone were watching and wondering what I was doing, whether I was taking drugs or had diarrhea. By now finding a bathroom had become a source of concern whenever I would travel.

When I settled down to catch some sleep, a group of teenagers gathered near the bathroom and spent the night laughing and joking. By the time we landed I was thoroughly exhausted. It was evening, and the wait for my connection seemed endless.

In the months before I left, I had experienced a brand new emotion for me: fear. All summer the questions ate at me. Could I handle such a long trip given my nights? Could I maintain such a restricted diet and be able to carry out days of research with a language I hadn't used since I was a teenager visiting my father at his home in Mexico City? I was also afraid of sharing the Mothers' grief and the avalanche of emotions that I knew would assail me upon my arrival.

I was uneasy too about the volatile political situation and the two attempted military coups the previous year. Although democratic government returned to Argentina after the military junta fell in 1984, the military retained an important political power, the security police were still ubiquitous, and the future was uncertain. My husband asked me, "Do you really need to take such a trip?" I answered him, "absolutely," denying my apprehension. Nor did I tell him about the telephone call to my senator and his response through an aide: "You are traveling at your own risk." Since my illness was so new, I didn't know how to speak of it or how to share my concerns. I was also wary of voicing them, not wanting to be dissuaded. I was in deep denial.

I arrived in Buenos Aires the next day at noon, worried about how I would recognize the Mothers and how I would have the strength to make the last leg of the trip to the hotel. But when I stepped into the crowded waiting room of the Buenos Aires airport, I recognized two elderly women with white head scarves as the Mothers. As I opened my arms and ran toward them, I noticed with astonishment how the waiting crowds edged away from the Mothers in fear.

All I could think of was a shower and rest, but as we climbed into the bus for the journey into Buenos Aires, Juana de Pargament, a tiny woman in her midseventies with the movements and energy of a dancer, told me that the Mothers were having a very important meeting I must attend. Mercedes Mereño, another one of the Mothers, accompanied Juana. It was some time before I realized that this was not just a courtesy but also a form of protection.

Their office was a shock: I stared at huge posters with photos of their "disappeared" children, hundreds of young people smiling at me from the wall, who had been tortured and killed in 365 clandestine concentration camps on the pretext that they were guerrilla terrorists. My stomach lurched, and I was incapable of words. Having shown me their reason for being, Juana and Mercedes ushered me into the room where the Mothers were meeting and where they greeted me with welcoming smiles. They waited for me to speak, but I was still digesting the vision of all the "disappeared" children. I smiled back at the Mothers and managed to greet them, then listened in silence to a heated discussion about preparing a press release on President Alfonsin's lack of firmness with the military.

It was some hours before Juana accompanied me to my hotel, where I collapsed into bed. I put off seeing the Mothers until the following day in order to recover somewhat and to gather my wits. I felt disoriented in a country that combined a democratic facade with features of a police state. In fact, I was entering two completely alien territories at the same time: the unknown province of my illness, and a society fraught with hidden dangers.

These experiences would be intertwined for the next seven years of my life. At the time, I thought I was learning about the Mothers' unusual political organization. In fact, I was simultaneously beginning to face the fear and anguish of a debilitating illness, for I wrestled with my stamina and ultimately with a new, searing pain during my time with the Mothers. I also discovered how I could feel so many different emotions simultaneously: anguish, rage, and the exhilaration of witnessing their bravery. I thought it was a moment in time, but my stay with them was an introduction to the endless turmoil of living with IC. It would be punctuated with joy when I finished a piece of writing or could sleep without pain. The perpetual weaving and reweaving of powerful feelings was not only part of my experience in Argentina; it was (and is) the typical weather in the country of chronic conditions, like massive cumulus clouds forming and re-forming above a mountain.

I was not completely at sea in this new setting, because of my experiences with my father when I was young. His bizarre ways of exposing me to new cultures helped me to navigate the strange political landscape in Argentina. He felt uncomfortable in the United States from the time we first emigrated there, and when I was ten years old he left the United States, spending the rest of his life in various parts of Mexico, of Chile, and in Lima, Peru, and São Paulo, Brazil, before returning to Paris when he was elderly. I stayed with him in Mexico and São Paulo, and for a period in Lima with friends of his when I was a teenager.

Instead of giving me guidance to help me in such new and different environments, he insisted I cope on my own. Although I didn't realize it at the time, this would be one of the most important lessons I would carry with me both when I became ill and when I traveled to Argentina. As soon as I arrived in Mexico, he announced: "Americans are hated in these countries because they live in enclaves and don't mingle. While you are here, you won't speak English and you'll learn the language." I did learn a halting Spanish while listening to my father speak with his colleagues. I also learned to love a city I wandered through for hours with one of his colleague's mistresses. My father knew little about children or how to be a parent, so he simply treated me as an adult although I was eleven at the time, ferrying me to his evening outings with his business friends. I nursed the whiskey sours he ordered for me and listened to their conversations, absorbing a language and also a culture while getting a glimpse of the seamier side of politics as I heard his associates speak of "their senator."

When I visited him in São Paulo a few years later, my father greeted me with his favorite phrase: "Learn the language, get to know the people." Since he was at work during the day, my lessons consisted of listening to the radio and taking the trolley from one end of the city to another at his suggestion. I can still hear the advertisement for pineapples bursting out of his small radio, "Abacaxi Elephante!" and the haunting Brazilian music. Learning the rudiments of a new language was not difficult. Picking up new customs by trial and error proved more daunting as I found myself saying the wrong things when we visited his friends. Over and over again, my father would challenge me to navigate the unknown.

Thus, when I arrived in Buenos Aires, I knew how to blend into a new culture and to learn quickly and on my feet. I spent my days with the Mothers in their office, which was actually a house called the "Mothers' House." I had never seen a place like this, with a kitchen where the Mothers cooked their own lunches and ate them on hastily cleared desks. In late afternoon they cooked dinners for the young people who arrived after work or school to help them prepare for marches and demonstrations and to work on their newspapers. One of the Mothers, Susana da Guidano, would pick up her shopping bag at a quarter of twelve every day just to buy some chicken to accommodate my restricted diet, something the Mothers could ill afford. Like the other Mothers, she had no difficulty combining her political forays with tender caring. In that warren of rooms, the Mothers were typically greeting visitors and journalists from abroad, having a conference with their lawyers, who were also volunteers, and writing press releases, all simultaneously. Once, I saw Susana hastily pull out a sewing machine and create a banner for that day's march.

As my illness worsened, I would see this fusion of their work and lives as an important marker in the remaking of my own unstructured days. It seemed as if the Mothers were living in chaos while they were actually accomplishing a great deal. In later years my friends would remark on how much I was doing, but they neither saw nor understood the unpredictability and strangeness of my schedule; I often worked an hour or two before dawn and rested during the day. Like the Mothers' days, each of my days would be different. I would have to learn how to seize any moment to pick up the threads of my projects.

On weekends, when the Mothers' office was closed and the city shut down, I strolled the streets of Buenos Aires, awed by the scale of this city, avenues as broad as football fields divided by lush greenery. The architecture seemed European, but the size of the buildings and the open spaces reminded me that this was the country of vast pampas. But most of the time I remained in my hotel room exhausted from my work.

As I walked the streets, I would soon learn that nothing was what it seemed. My fear about my stamina was mirrored by a new fear for my physical safety. Mornings when I walked to the Mothers' House on Yrigoyen Street, I routinely passed schoolchildren dressed in uniforms and people rushing to work. After a while I began to notice this city's layers of reality, the lines snaking around the corner with people desperate to withdraw their savings after currency devaluations and the number of police in the poorer neighborhoods. From the Mothers' window, I witnessed police beating up disabled people who had gathered for a demonstration. They were accustomed to using the sidewalks to set up market stands as a way of earning their living, a privilege that had recently been revoked by the government. As they lined up in wheelchairs and with their canes, the police suddenly swooped down on them, hitting out right and left with truncheons and wounding many of these people, who collapsed on the pavement. I gasped in horror and disbelief.

On my first Thursday in Buenos Aires, I accompanied the Mothers on their weekly pilgrimage to demonstrate in the huge Plaza de Mayo before the presidential palace, as they had done since the early days of the junta to demand information about their children. It was raining heavily. There were not many people milling around, but I noticed police cars circling the plaza with video cameras thrust through their open windows. The president of the Mothers' organization, Hebe de Bonafini, an imposing woman with a vitriolic tongue, picked up the microphone and boomed through it, "Today we have a special visitor with us, Margarita Bouvard from Boston." I was terrified, realizing I was being videotaped and remembering the conversation with the warning from my senator's aide: "At your own risk." It was the first of many such unsettling experiences with the security police tailing the Mothers.

When the Mothers would leave for their weekly march in the plaza, they would suddenly become silent, donning their white scarves and gathering together in a phalanx. They were united not only by purpose but also for mutual protection. In my second week with the Mothers, I saw the police try to drag off one of the Mothers' young supporters as they circled the obelisk in the middle of the plaza. I gasped as the diminutive Juana de Pargament reared up before the policeman, shaking her finger at him and yelling, "Take your hands off that kid." Surprisingly, the man complied.

Juana and I become very close. She was able to speak some English and, given my broken Spanish, became the person who would answer my questions the most frequently. One Sunday afternoon she invited me for tea in her home, which was not far from the Mothers' House. I entered a spacious and sunny living room where we sat and talked about her grandchildren from her daughter. Then she said, "Now I will show you something," and opened the door to a dark and musty room. "It was my son's medical office," she told me. Fifteen years after the military had dragged him away, everything was still in place: his array of medical books, his desk, and his instruments. "There was always a long line of people waiting for him, those who could pay and many who could not. He never turned anyone away, " Juana continued. I was speechless, imagining a son like my own who is socially progressive and takes pleasure in volunteering his time. The absence tore at my heart. I envisioned Juana passing this door several times a day and reliving her son's "disappearance."

There were times when my illness seemed to take a backseat in my astonishment at the bravery of these women and my realization of the dangers of being a dissident in this country. I was too absorbed adapting to this new environment. Their children reminded me of my own, of my students, and of all the young people I worked with and loved. My feelings as a mother, my outrage at what had happened to the "disappeared," and my growing affection for these women overwhelmed me. Because they had been infiltrated in the past, it had been very difficult to get them to agree to my visit, but now that I was with them, they gathered me in as if I was one of them.

Mornings, I called room service for tea to conserve my energy and to work on my notes. But one morning I noticed that the waiter was a new one and looked like a thug, an agent of the security police, staring at my notes. Before I left, I carefully stuffed them under the mattress.

As I shared the Mothers' days with them and interviewed their young supporters as well as the psychiatrists and other social activists who worked with them, my political beliefs that I had accumulated over the years—the value of a political democracy as opposed to socialism or communism—didn't seem to apply. I wondered whether, if I lived here and had no other frame of reference, I would be so angered by social conditions that I would become a leftist inclined toward the kind of democratic socialism that existed in Sweden. In the years to come, all my personal views about the importance of a career and the attendant recognition would also be undermined as I tried to re-create a life for myself around the limitations interstitial cystitis imposed on me.

The Mothers and their supporters would become role models of courage as I struggled against a physical condition that threatened to overwhelm me. Hebe de Bonafini, the president of the organization, had barely finished a grammar school education and never stepped out of the role of stay-at-home housewife until her two sons were kidnapped by the security police and killed in concentration camps. She was oblivious to her safety and not only spoke loudly at any political gathering where she was definitely not welcome but also became adept at outwitting the powerful government and the security forces, anticipating their moves. For example, the night before a military parade, she directed her young supporters to paint the word "assassins" all along the route they would be taking.

When her oldest son, Jorge, "disappeared" she stepped out of the known security of her house and into a terrifying world. She and her husband traveled all over the country contacting friends, trying to find her son. Then, when she was waiting in line outside a police station hoping for news of his whereabouts, she noticed other women and began talking to them. They told her they had begun meeting and asked her to join them. The night before doing so, she could hardly sleep for her terror and uncertainty, for any type of gathering was prohibited and severely punished at the time. Attending the meeting of the Mothers was the beginning of a complete transformation of her life, from that of a private, retiring woman into that of a woman who spent her time organizing, demonstrating, and speaking out, revealing a gift for acerbic language as she designed the Mothers' yearly slogans. During what is now called the "Dirty War" she also lost her son Jorge's pregnant wife and her younger son. Soon after, her husband died of cancer, and she and her daughter were all that remained of an affectionate and close family. By then she felt she had nothing to lose except her own life and dedicated it to the cause of calling the military leaders to account. She not only would become a nationally recognized leader but would receive awards from human rights foundations throughout Europe.

The week before my trip, there had been another of many attempts on her life. A car had zoomed up the sidewalk in front of her house in the city of La Plata, fifty miles outside Buenos Aires, intending to smash her against the wall, but somehow she escaped. On the tenth day of my stay, Hebe turned to me and said, "I want you to come to La Plata with me. I'm going to give a talk at the university there tomorrow morning." Then she looked me over. "So you'd better go back to your hotel and rest right now because we are leaving at one a.m."

Before my rest, I called the American consulate to report my plans in case something should happen and my husband was unable to trace me. The person at the other end of the line didn't bother taking any of the information but simply replied, "Have a good trip," and hung up. That was yet another shock, for although our government was officially critical of the former junta, I had yet to learn about the collusion of our own military, which had trained Argentine soldiers in torture techniques.

When Hebe and I set off for the bus station, I was frankly terrified both for my safety and for my stamina. During the ride, while Hebe was loudly holding forth about politics, I noticed two men watching and listening across the aisle. "Hebe," I said, "We're being spied on." "So what?" she retorted. "Let them learn something."

I was so worn out by the trip that I slept until noon the following day, missing out on the university presentation. I was disappointed because I wanted very much to see Hebe address the students and speak to their fear at a university where whole classes of students had "disappeared." I did manage to march with the Mothers in La Plata and to have tea with them afterward. Their numbers were smaller and fewer followers accompanied them here than in Buenos Aries, but the march had a dignity and sobriety that impressed me. I noticed that, midway, one of the fathers slipped into the march to accompany the Mothers and saw the grief etched on his quiet face. As usual, their demonstration was surrounded by a heavy police presence.

Afterward they were laughing and talking, celebrating the birth of a grandchild to one Mother's daughter living in exile in Spain and passing around the bitter mate drink I developed a taste for. When the electricity sputtered and finally failed, they barely noticed. At the time, I was surprised by the juxtaposition of danger and joy, but as the years passed I found myself able to savor moments of intense pleasure during the darkest periods of pain and sleeplessness.

All through my stay in Buenos Aries, I was learning from the Mothers and from their supporters too. One of these was an artist, Carmen d'Elia, who had been with them from the very beginning, sharing their triumphs and also the dangers of facing the ubiquitous security police. During the time of the junta, she slept in a different location every night because she knew the army was after her for her reformist views. She asked me if I was a *militante*, meaning a political activist. I tried to explain my volunteer activities, but hers was a world in which the political was primary; whether or not one took a moral stand defined the way she related to people. She lived frugally on the sale of her paintings and her teaching, supporting two teenage sons. Neither her family situation nor the dangers she courted could sway her from accompanying the Mothers on their demonstrations or helping them to make posters. As I pored over the photo documents tracing the history of the Mothers' organization, Carmen was always there with them.

Although our experiences and our cultures were so different, Carmen and I had many long conversations over coffee when the Mothers' office shut down in late afternoon. Once she confided, "One day I passed the Mothers' demonstration in the Plaza and suddenly I felt hope. I was suffering from cancer at the time. When I decided to join them during the most terrible days of the dictatorship it was if I had stepped out of the prison of despair." I would remember that statement when I too felt as if my IC imprisoned me. I discovered that continuing to write in order to awaken people to the problems and also the triumphs of living with illness—and addressing groups on such taboo subjects—would open windows and doors in my life, making me feel less powerless.

My list of publications and years of teaching suddenly seemed of little account. I was the one who was learning, not only about politics and women's roles, but also about the broader issues of courage and priorities in life. Evenings in my hotel, while pondering a sea of handwritten notes to myself, I realized that the guidelines I had carefully constructed to conduct my research didn't apply to the Mothers' reality. I would have to begin from ground zero. This searching would help me to redefine the life I had constructed as someone who enjoyed good health and to realize that, in order to grow, I had to continually reassess my perspectives and my values, a painful but ultimately liberating process. For example, I discovered that my concern for people in difficulties and for social justice, which had always been part of my life, was as valuable if not more so than the socially recognized career I would soon have to give up. I would learn that I still could accomplish much of social value despite my truncated days and limited stamina.

The Mothers' sorrow affected me so deeply that I began marching with them during their nighttime demonstrations and experiencing their anger with my whole being. One night when Maria del Rosario de Cerurrti was lining up the Mothers in preparation for a march, I joined them in the front line instead of going back to the hotel. She looked at me with surprise. I had stepped out of the role of a woman conducting research and joined the Mothers' efforts, which I continued to participate in during the rest of my stay. The anger I absorbed from them was an important lesson, for my religious upbringing as well as my socialization had instilled in me the attitude that women who expressed anger were just "bitches."

This experience would help me learn how to acknowledge the rage I felt at my illness as I fumed at my shortened days and all that I would have to forgo because of my diminished energy, at my interrupted nights that left me exhausted, at the loss of a known world. I also chafed at the indifference to my condition that many people conveyed, and at their lack of understanding. I lived in a turbulence of outrage, fear, and sorrow for the "disappeared" and also for my changing circumstances. The Mothers were teaching me an important lesson: that informed emotion was useful in addressing tragic circumstances.

During an evening demonstration, I began to understand the seeming safety of indifference and the public's fear of these women. We were marching ten abreast down the streets, and I was in the first row of demonstrators among the Mothers. We were accompanied by hundreds of supporters carrying the Mothers' banners and shouting, "Apparicion con vida!" (Bring back the disappeared alive!). But as we passed through the busy streets, people slipped inside; shutters and doors slammed shut. It seemed as if the foreign television cameras were the only ones aware of us. It felt eerie: a whole country wanting to make the Mothers invisible.

Later, as my illness took hold, I too would learn about invisibility from the conversations that flowed around me. I often listened to friends talking about their many activities, while the hurdles I faced daily were greeted by embarrassed silence. I felt like an alien as they spoke of jogging and keeping fit. I tried to convey the struggles of my everyday life in words that would explain but not alarm or alienate people, but I discovered that it is as difficult for a healthy person to imagine the constraints I endure as it is for someone who lives in a tropical climate to imagine shoveling snow on a January morning. We were unable to converse about my new life simply because it was so different from the lives of healthy people. Our reference points were so diverse that we could have been living in separate cultures even though we shared the same landscape.

I understood perfectly when a close friend of mine who had recently undergone surgery and chemotherapy for breast cancer told me that she was unable to speak about her experiences. "I try to put out feelers," she said, and "they are not taken up. It's as if nothing ever happened to me. I feel as if I am alone somewhere while the world passes me by." Yet another friend would tell me, "Once you're diagnosed with cancer, you're put in another world, you're outside." Thus reentering society as a person who was ill would become a major effort for me.

But now, in this new setting, I was quick to learn about political parties and factions in Argentina, about the gulf in this society between those who told the truth and those who maintained a deliberate blindness, refusing to face political realities. I was with the Mothers while they received threatening phone calls from the police, but many Argentines wanted to believe that democracy had returned. They wanted to forget the past horrors under the junta and ignore the continuing presence of the torturers.

It would take me years of struggling with illness to understand that to find the truth is also to descend into the chaos of our feelings. I would discover that we must not only allow these emotions but also ignore social mores that want to restrict their expression so as not to alarm or offend or awaken us to a deeper reality. But at the time, I was so passionate about what I was experiencing that I paid insufficient heed to my illness despite being very tired and needing to rest before evening demonstrations. I vowed to postpone the book on women and human rights and instead write the Mothers' story.

A few days before I left Buenos Aires, knifelike pains in my bladder prevented me from sleeping at night. The urgency to urinate still awakened me every hour or two, but the pains came like lightning when my bladder was empty. I felt as if it was being torn apart, leaving me aghast and bewildered. I thought these nightly bouts of pain must be an aberration, but when I returned home they became the norm.

Did my stay in Buenos Aires, where I pushed the limits of my endurance, worsen my condition? Perhaps it did. But the book-writing project I began there would hold me together during the harrowing years when I tried to make a life for myself. It was also the very first instance of a new working style I developed that substituted intensity for length. My trip lasted two weeks. I could not have managed a longer period given my condition, but in that short time I lived years and with a new depth. It was a prelude to using the one or two hours I felt well on a good day as if they were the long hours healthy people enjoy. As my illness became more acute, the pattern of long months when I was unable to do much, punctuated by short bursts of travel or writing, would become my "new normal."

I returned a changed person in many ways. I couldn't stop talking to my husband about what I had seen in Argentina, as if by repeating my experiences I could understand them more clearly. I was brimming with a psychic energy that was fueled by outrage. But I had to put away my notes to begin the new semester at college. The grief I brought home with me for what had happened to the Mothers' children unexpectedly served as a foreshadowing of all the raw feelings of living with a debilitating condition.

✻ ✻ ✻

The fall of 1989, I struggled to get through the days with little sleep. It never occurred to me that I wasn't going to improve, that I couldn't keep up my brimming life. I had never been seriously ill before, and because none of the physicians I consulted had given me any guidelines for living with IC, it was easy to remain in denial, an emotion that happens to dominate the first of the five stages of grieving. Although my illness would have no calendar of diagnosis, treatment, and cure, my reaction to it would indeed follow the phases a person experiences after a loss.

In October I received a call for papers for a spring conference on women and leadership organized by the Cherokee Nation in Talequah, Oklahoma. Ordinarily I would have turned it down given my condition, but I applied on a whim because it would give me an opportunity to present a paper about the Mothers. I had to call ahead and request a special diet and a quiet room, but at the time I believed that I still had enough energy to attend such a gathering.

Oddly enough, this conference would provide me with yet another important learning experience. At my college I was teaching European Governments as well as International Relations. Neither my work with the Mothers nor such a conference had any relevance to these subjects.

Thus, when I arrived in Talequah, I once again found myself learning about a new culture in compressed time, and thus, once again, my illness actually gave me an opportunity to range further than I would have been able to do in my current job. While I felt that my world was changing beyond recognition because of my extreme fatigue, another one seemed to be opening up that would absorb me for years to come. By hindsight, these two trips, to Argentina and Oklahoma, turned out to be special gifts that would guide me through my illness.

The conference was a revelation to me. At the airport I met a friendly blonde woman who identified herself as a member of the Nation. Startled, I asked her to explain. She replied that she was one-sixteenth Cherokee and thus given the option to remain a member. She and her husband were eager to do so because "we have children and I know they would be very well cared for by the People if anything happened to us." I had more to learn at this gathering where I was a minority in a totally different culture. It awakened me to a set of values that would help me address my illness, since the Cherokee live with a deep reverence for life in all its manifestations. That outlook inspired me to begin reading about Native American spirituality as I struggled for meaning in my new situation.

Unfortunately my requests for a special diet went unheeded, and I had to scramble to find something to eat at each meal. What I once considered small matters loomed large in my daily life. One evening, we were treated to a sumptuous banquet of Native American foods that I could participate in only by watching.

At an afternoon session on women and spirituality, I met the presenter, a Cherokee poet and writer, Awiakta, and as we talked afterward, I struck up a friendship with this imposing person with raven hair and a ready laugh. We spent the following afternoon together, sharing our thoughts as if we had known each other all our lives. As I stared in perplexity at a silver pendant she wore around her neck, a deer leaping within an atom, she told me "Awiakta means little deer in Cherokee. My father worked on a secret project for the Atomic Energy Commission in Oak Ridge, Tennessee, where we lived when I was a child, so I lived in two worlds." Thus, she introduced me to the Cherokee concept of compromise and inclusion. We discussed our beliefs on the importance of cooperation, mutuality, and caring in society. Both of us felt that a spirituality that didn't inform personal and social relations with deep respect was of little value. I was filled with admiration for the way in which she carried out her work on behalf of her people, without any self-promotion.

In that short period of time, she introduced me to a culture in which older women have primary roles, and to a way of life with differing views of time, history, and ethics.

Neither of us could have guessed that, years later, she and I would spend hours on the telephone talking about her bout with cancer and my illness and that I would devote a chapter to her and other Native American women in the book I ultimately wrote about women and human rights.

This experience in Talequah would provide me with the seeds of new perspectives. They would lie dormant while I reconstructed my daily life, but would ultimately become an increasingly important strand in new ways of considering empowerment. The Native American women who organized the event made clear that women had power in their nation and therefore didn't need to speak of how to acquire it. Just like the Mothers of the Plaza de Mayo, they combined political savvy with caring ways, for they too had learned to survive in a prejudiced and hostile world. I too would learn to recognize that I was not without resources despite a debilitating illness.

Unfortunately, my presentation was scheduled for the evening at the very last session of the conference. I spent the whole day in my room, resting and overpreparing. By now I was so wracked by lack of proper sleep that I no longer trusted my memory and was unable to give talks with spontaneity. On the day of the presentation, I cut my talk considerably because I was fatigued.

Little by little, my life was becoming more problematic. I was now spending much thought and emotional energy to just get through the ordinary events of a day. In fact, this would prove to be the last time I could attend such a conference. But while I no longer enjoyed the ease of the healthy, I still wanted to be engaged with the world. Thus I lived with contradictions, and contradictory feelings: anger at having to spend so much of my energy doing what most people take for granted, and exhilaration when I managed to go beyond that and give a lecture.

In what seemed like such a short period, I had entered two different worlds that had much to teach me. While eager to learn more about cultures that drew on values I also cherished, I was caught in what seemed to me a constantly shrinking world where the slightest physical efforts, such as participating in a social event that lasted for more than two hours, or running a simple errand, or finding a bathroom, became problems to solve.

4

A WORLD WITHOUT MARKERS

AT THE END of the semester in 1989, I could no longer keep up my frenetic schedule and made an appointment to see the president of my college. I wanted to scale back my teaching load so I could hold on to my career. It seemed strange to be sitting in that office and asking if I could drop one of my three courses while keeping all the duties of a full-time professor, such as committees and student advising. "Marguerite," she replied, "you've been with us for a long time," agreeing to my request—a response that surprised me, for we had frequently been at loggerheads over her treatment of faculty and students. She had made it publicly clear that she didn't care for me, because I asked so many pointed questions during faculty meetings; I never realized that she actually valued my contributions. I believed that this lessening of my responsibilities would allow me to keep on teaching, to continue my life as before.

That January, in the break between semesters, I traveled to the Virginia Center for the Creative Arts, an artists' retreat I visited yearly to work on my poetry. Even though the Center is not equipped for special meals, the cook made a heroic effort to accommodate me. Luckily my studio had a cot where I could nap afternoons. The wonderful feature of the Center is the utter privacy. No one is supposed to visit another studio without express invitation, so I had the luxury of not having to measure myself against people who had no physical hurdles to face. I had two weeks of solitude there and could follow my own schedule and work at my own pace. Despite my condition, poems about the Mothers came pouring out; I finally had an opportunity to process my stay with the Mothers and give voice to the terrible sorrow that my time there had awakened. I wept copiously over the fate of the Mothers' children as I wrote, and over the lives of the Mothers haunted by such a wrenching loss. I now realize that I was also expressing my frustration and grief over my condition even though it was buried so deeply.

When I returned, my teaching mirrored my fatigue. My classes used to hum with excitement. I had felt as if I were bringing the world to students who rarely left the country, much less the state of Massachusetts. I had them read African novels so they could have a better grasp of conditions abroad, and I remember how voluble my students suddenly became as we discussed these works. I created panel discussions so that my students, who had been brought up in a Catholic tradition and were often too compliant, could debate and disagree, something they learned to do with fervor. "What's the right response to President Mugabe's new laws?" a student would ask, and I would reply, "You decide." Because the college had no financial resources for activities in support of teaching, I often felt like a tour guide, bringing students to exotic lands such as Harvard or M.I.T where an international leader was speaking or to foreign films as I urged them to become familiar with issues in the world. Once I brought my poetry students to a mobbed theater at Harvard to hear Czeslaw Milosz, who had just received the Nobel Prize for Poetry. "Dr. Bouvard, why are we here?" they asked. "Just listen. You are in the presence of greatness, and someday you will remember this," I told them.

Previously my seminars would sometimes run beyond the allotted period as the students would heatedly discuss issues that touched on feminism. "When do you think we could finally have a woman president?" I once asked them, and that began a long exchange. Once I divided my theory seminar into two groups to have them discuss a recent case in a small suburb outside Chicago where a judge, ruling in favor of the American Civil Liberties Union, had allowed a group of neo-Nazis to hold a march in a predominantly Jewish neighborhood. I wanted my students to understand the complexities of free speech and ethics. They argued long and hard without reaching a conclusion. They were learning about uncertainty and the difficulties of choice. I then had them read Hitler's *Mein Kampf* and asked them to circle words that had a visceral appeal before reading for content. "Why?" one of my students asked. "Because you'll understand how political leaders frame their speeches to get mass appeal," I replied.

Now, as I read the students' evaluations of my political theory seminar, I was devastated by a complaint that I had ended the seminar ten minutes before the usual closing, for I was convinced that nobody had noticed the changes in my style. I was straining to keep up my pace, and I had little perspective on how I was exacerbating my illness by pushing myself beyond my limits. Part of me was convinced that my former life was just around the corner, waiting for me to step onto it like a carousel. But deep inside, I knew that I would have to make significant changes in my life. The prospect was disorienting and deeply upsetting.

I kept making myself lists of action items as if I were still in charge. I spent more time writing in my journal, with the very first page of the new year devoted to planning my future, mulling over alternatives. I noted that I would like to continue working two-thirds instead of full time and that I would like to design a seminar on human rights. I even dreamed of working for Amnesty International, interviewing people who had just fled their country. A close friend of my niece Michele was a lawyer for Amnesty International and a possible contact. Or perhaps I might teach only the poetry workshops, which meant so much to me. The page bristled with possibilities, as if I could choose.

Meanwhile I continued bringing guest speakers on human rights into my classes because I wanted my students to understand that individuals are not powerless. A close friend of mine, Eva Brantley, was an international human rights lawyer who happened to be blind. With her guide dog, Waldo, in tow she would tell my class about establishing a union for child laborers in India or her clandestine visits to Myanmar to take evidence of the mistreatment of the indigenous peoples there. Ironically, I was trying to raise my students' awareness of their own possibilities while it seemed as if I was losing my grip on everything familiar in my universe. I could no longer control the way I navigated the day and felt like the captain of a ship passing through dangerous shoals and rocks, needing to stay alert to the smallest details. What had once been normal undertakings such as writing new lectures or attending meetings were now so taxing that I had to stop and consider whether I could do them.

When the spring semester ended in May 1990, I took a sabbatical leave. Surprisingly, the president of my college expressed the hope that I would return renewed in 1991. I was foolish enough to share that optimism.

That fall I had a fellowship at the Wellesley College Center for Research on Women, where I planned to begin my research on Argentina, for my expertise was in European governments. I found myself sitting through the weekly seminars, where the scholars would present their research, in a state I can only describe as jet lag. I'd been up so much of the night that I had difficulty focusing, talking, or remembering. The lively discussions swirling around me seemed distant and alien. Although this headachy, drugged feeling became a frequent part of my life, I doggedly attended most sessions.

Since I had no other obligations there than to pursue my own project, I was burning to fly back to Buenos Aires and the Mothers, not only to complete my research, but also simply because I wanted to be with them. We had forged very close bonds during my last stay, and I felt a deep love for each one of them. By now I needed long afternoon naps, and the slightest effort tired me. Again I wrestled with the wisdom of such a step and whether I could handle it. It was not only my health that would be at stake but my safety, for at the time there had already been an attempted military coup and the possibility of another was immanent.

Once while sitting in my usual late afternoon hour of meditation, a practice I had begun in earnest that year to help me sort out the turbulence of my feelings, an image came to my mind that helped me with my decision. In that image I was standing in a crowded subway, holding on to a strap. When I looked up, I noticed that the strap was hanging from a solid bar of light. That sight comforted me, making me feel that I would be able to manage in such a volatile political environment. I felt it was a sign that I should go ahead.

This time I was not completely unaware of what lay ahead for me. I didn't make a reservation in the hotel I had stayed in before, which was frequented by journalists and foreigners, but planned instead to find a small one in the business district, where I could remain anonymous and unobserved. I also made a very uncharacteristic purchase before I left, an expensive camera. I sensed that my time as a salaried professor was coming to an end, and I wanted to preserve the images of these remarkable older women. My son, who travels frequently, generously gave me a business-class ticket for a direct flight to Buenos Aires, so I was able to sleep on and off during this very long journey.

I left in early October, staying for two weeks and just missing another attempted military coup. By some miracle I experienced a remission, which not only carried me through my trip but also gave me a week to write unencumbered by symptoms. Granted, I was in bed by eight o'clock every evening, gray with exhaustion, but I completed my work of interviewing the Mothers as well as poring over the Mothers' documents with a fierce intensity. This time, I knew I would have to spend weekends in

complete rest and brought some pieces of hand quilting I could turn to
when I didn't have energy for much else. I was learning how to fill the periods of solitude my condition imposed on me.

The decision to interview the Mothers was a challenging one, for my
illness had stripped me of any protective borders; I knew their grief
would become mine. Hebe set aside a private room for me, and over a
few days I spent more than an hour with each of about a dozen mothers.
Evel Astrabe de Petrini, an effervescent and beautiful blonde woman in
her early fifties, told me "I was home alone with my two sons when the
doorbell rang. My husband was away on a job. When I answered the
door there were ten heavily armed men in front of me. They told me they
were looking for a thief in the neighborhood and then asked me if I was
alone. They then dragged my two sons on the ground and began kicking
them in the genitals. They held them at gunpoint while they searched the
house, pillaging. Then one of them asked me which one of my sons was
Sergio—they were going to take him away. I was terrified and pleaded
with them. 'He's done nothing, take me instead.' But they dragged him
away. He was only eighteen." I was shocked and found myself holding
her close in silent sympathy.

"My son was beaten up by the security police right in front of his own
children before they dragged him away, " Susana da Guidano told me.
"He was a world-renowned nuclear physicist so letters came pouring in
on his behalf from around the world, but they failed to save him." I wept
with her and embraced her, learning how telling one's painful story is a
way of healing. I was releasing my own unexpressed and submerged grief,
the loss of myself to this illness. That sorrow made me adept at drawing the Mothers out and hearing their hair-raising experiences. Susana's
daughter-in-law came to the office so that I could talk to her as well. Again
we cried and held each other. "Thank you for wanting to know about
me," she said before leaving, a statement that would resonate in the coming years, when many people demonstrated that they would rather not
know about what I was experiencing.

I realized that by telling their stories the Mothers were assuaging their
grief and that I too would need to share my lesser trials and to be listened
to with understanding rather than fear. I was not only gathering material
for my book; I was learning a difficult but powerful language of truthfulness that many healthy people find hard to hear.

That this truthfulness could be expressed publicly was also a revelation. One morning a young woman arrived at the Mothers' office in tears

because the police had dragged her husband away and she could find no trace of him at the police station. To my surprise, the Mothers encouraged her to go immediately to the Plaza de Mayo, take up the microphone, and tell the crowd what had happened, which she did with passion. I listened to her shout out "They came for my husband in the middle of the night when we were asleep and beat him up in front of me. Then they dragged him away. I want to know where he is. I want him back. This shouldn't be happening today," hearing such strength in her voice. Now I understand that the Mothers not only intended to publicize such abuses but also didn't want the woman to become silenced by fear. I would need years of work to break my own silence about my painful illness.

As I revisited the plaza on Thursdays I learned to recognize the plainclothesmen. One day I spotted one before me, sitting casually on a bench while scrutinizing passersby, and all at once I was swept by a searing rage. With sudden clarity I recognized that the fear that kept me wishing to remain unseen had infringed on my freedom, and my anger made me leap over that fear. I always carried my camera and for an instant felt like photographing him; instead I stared at him with a disgusted expression. I felt liberated. Women are not supposed to express anger in most cultures, but I learned that it could serve as a motor propelling me through my illness. Just as the anger over the ubiquitous presence of security police fired my work on the Mothers, anger over my increasing physical frailty helped me move through the chaos of my new condition.

The day of my departure there was trouble brewing. The labor unions had planned a big demonstration and the Mothers wanted to participate, both by criticizing the union bureaucracy and by supporting the workers with their huge banners. As we entered the plaza I saw policemen on the rooftops, their rifles pointing downward at the gathering demonstrators. Given their distance, this time I felt comfortable taking their pictures. Then suddenly I heard a cry: "Colonel Seneldein [a notorious torturer during the dark days of the military dictatorship] has entered the plaza." He was thought to be in prison but was now supposedly at liberty. Before I could blink, the plaza turned into a bloody melee with the police swinging their clubs rights and left. I was stunned, unable to move until Juana, who is half my size, grabbed my arm and yelled, "Corre [Run], Margarita, corre," as she pulled me away into the street.

Hebe de Bonafini saved the day by marching through the streets with a megaphone, chanting, "We have left the plaza because we do not wish to share it with a man like Colonel Seneldein." She held herself with dignity and strength while mobs of demonstrators swept past us toward the plaza. When we arrived at the Mothers' House, I was dazed and shaken. I had brought my suitcase there because I needed to leave for a flight a few hours later. The Mothers were calmly preparing tea as if it was an ordinary afternoon and I began eating pastries voraciously, something totally out of character, for I am very rarely hungry and don't like desserts.

Juana decided to take me to the airport in style, on a bus that made no stops and swished to the airport in an hour instead of the usual hour and forty-five minutes. As we settled ourselves, an American couple sat down in front of us surrounded by shopping bags. They were relaxed and pleased with their sightseeing and their visit, seemingly unaware of what was happening in this country. It made me think of how I myself had taken both my safety and my health so for granted that I rarely thought about them.

⁂

The rest of my year was spent trying to conduct research and organize the material I'd gathered in Argentina. I had brought back some of the Mothers' original documents of their founding and early years, important primary sources. At this point, I was still able to periodically spend time in libraries. But my work didn't happen in an orderly fashion. There were weeks on end when I was so fatigued I was unable to do anything. I worked in fits and starts, at odd moments, and for short periods of time. I no longer had what most people take for granted: a schedule.

I also engaged in less taxing projects during those weeks when my main effort was to climb the mountain of the everyday. When I purchased the camera for the trip to Argentina, I also bought a sewing machine; I am a quilt maker, and I knew I would need an absorbing occupation when I was going through my down times. I had an ancient Sears machine and decided to buy one that would permit me to realize more elaborate designs. This pastime had also been woven into my work, for during difficult periods I would drive to a fabric store to relieve my stress and grant space to my artistic bent. Now, just thinking about colors and designs was a way of enriching my daily life.

Often I didn't even bother to drive the mile and a half to the Wellesley College Center for Research on Women. But there was one session I attended that year that highlighted the transformation in my perspectives. The session was on moral reasoning and directed by a political science professor at Wellesley. She handed out a sheet of paper with a list of six people applying for a heart transplant, and we were to select one who we believed would qualify. I was the only one of the scholars who, rather than choosing a renowned medical researcher, selected a convicted felon who had become a peacemaker among inmates.

My illness had taught me that there are no hierarchies when it comes to either serving or expressing our humanity. I remembered watching a special television report on the elections and the homeless that included a former architect, a secretary who had lost her job, and a mentally ill man, each of them lost and lonely but also courageous in insisting that the homeless be included within the political system as voters. I recognized within each one of them my own vulnerability and my dilemma.

At this time, I was plunged into a phase of the grieving process known as disorganization and which follows denial: the end of the life one has carefully constructed and the entrance into a world without markers. I felt I was adrift, no longer a professor, or a professional, but a person is search of an identity. I ached for my former life and the ease I had so taken for granted.

The following January, I once again turned to my poetry, spending a few restorative weeks at the Virginia Center for the Creative Arts, near the Blue Ridge Mountains, to write. It was the luxury of having hours and hours of reflection in my studio without feeling I needed to be "working" that would ultimately help me regain my bearings. I didn't know then that this rumination was extremely important work in itself and would become a significant part of my new life. In the artists' library I found a poem by the Spanish poet Antonio Machado:

> Why call
> those random paths
> roads?
> Everyone who walks
> walks
> like Jesus
> on water.

And a poem by the German poet Nelly Sachs:

> And the planets
> are born
> of the magic substances of pain.

Reading and writing in my journal, observing the fields outside my window, taking stock of what was good in my life—these became threads in my struggle to understand the physical and emotional changes I was experiencing. At the time, there was no public space for the private struggles of prolonged illness, and there was no one with whom I could share my confusion. I felt as if I was in a caesura, nowhere recognizable and surely lost. I wrote in my journal: *This illness is one of the most profound and challenging experiences of my life because it is a daily battle not only to confront it but also to prevent it from smothering love, poetry, friendship. The meadows opening outside my window, the distant mountains' blue lines and the huge clouds drifting past remind me that we too are always changing.* I began to sketch a few poems about living with illness that would over time become a new book project. I had always written about people caught in world events in my poetry, but now I began to portray my nights: *I am delivered into morning / with the stark vocabulary / of night, the lamp's red eye, / the body fisted over its pain /.* I lived in my own war zone.

As my sabbatical drew to a close, I noted in my journal: *After another painful night, my plan for new work at the college doesn't look so good this morning.* And finally, *Resolutions: 1. Contact publisher with a book plan. 2. Find a publisher for book of poems about the Mothers. 3. Place chapters in scholarly journals. 4. Apply for total disability.*

⁕⁕⁕

In the spring of 1991, I made an appointment with the president of my college to tell her I would not be returning. It was an extremely painful decision; it meant giving up the teaching that was so central to my life, ending twenty-five years of work at the college, and leaving a group of close colleagues. The meeting was brief and to the point. My statement to the president was accepted with a request that I put my intention in writing. As I walked out of her office, I felt as if I were diving into an empty swimming pool.

Afterward I kept saying to myself, "This is not really happening to me." I was devastated and felt as if some mechanical force was propelling me through a changing landscape. As I walked through halls filled with the swirl and chatter of students hurrying between classes, several of my colleagues waved as they rushed past with bulging briefcases. I had warm relations with several members of the staff, from the young woman who ran the administrative services in the lower floor to the academic dean's secretary, who was the rock of that office, to my dear friend Lily, who was the head of acquisitions in the library, but this was no longer my world.

Over the weekend, my husband and I drove to the college with an assortment of large boxes to begin the task of taking down the photographs and emptying my desk and the bookshelves in my office. As I carefully sorted the books, planning to leave quite a few behind for the department, it seemed as if I was packing a life into a few cartons.

I stored the boxes of course notes, articles, and journals in the attic because I couldn't bear to look at what seemed like shreds of my life. I wanted to throw them away, typical of my hastiness, but my husband insisted that I keep them, that I might need them sometime.

I missed my students and recalled how prescient I was, my last semester, in taping each one reading her poetry in the workshop I taught. My illness had changed me from the very demanding political science professor I once was, with my long reading lists, making me more sensitive to the pressures students faced. The night before a difficult examination I drove to the college to give the students a guided meditation and help them relax, something I would never have dreamed of doing before.

My department chair organized a party for me later that fall with a number of my favorite students and my closest colleagues. Three of them read testimonials they had written, and one of my students read a poem. I was glad I came, having considered calling to say I couldn't make it as I didn't feel up to it physically. One of my closest colleagues, Louise Lopman, also arranged a farewell dinner for me at a local restaurant. Eight of my friends from the college were there and presented me with a beautifully bound edition of a poetry book.

However, feelings don't always appear in tandem with events. Despite these touching farewells, I continued to dream that I was in the classroom, that I was preparing a syllabus for the new semester. At that point I felt that in my mind I would always be a professor. I was unwilling to let go.

∗ ∗ ∗

After submitting my resignation, the next step was to apply for disability. It was some kind of miracle that I had actually signed up for the group disability program at the college. The year before I became ill, I ran into the president's assistant as I was walking to one of my classes. She stopped me, saying she wanted to talk to me. I was surprised because the last time

I had spoken to her was some years before, when she was newly widowed and I'd brought her flowers. "Marguerite," she told me, "you haven't signed up for disability." "No, I haven't," I replied. "Why should I?" I had never been seriously ill before, and such insurance seemed somehow irrelevant. She was insistent in a very kind way, so I completed the forms little suspecting how grateful I would be in just a year.

The head of the personnel office at the college was a former student of mine. She started me on the application process and put me in touch with the insurance company. The company's administrator in charge of long-term disability informed me that I needed to begin with the Social Security office and that my payments were contingent on receiving Social Security.

I called for an appointment feeling as if I was somehow transformed, and soon I was sitting in the Framingham Social Security office with my husband. No longer wearing a suit or carrying a briefcase, I felt like an anonymous person. The office was seedy. I immediately felt the dividing line between the people patiently waiting for their appointments and the authority of the government officials behind their desks. Though I always believed that social standing meant nothing to me, I was now keenly aware that I had tumbled to the bottom of the social ladder and was almost in the position of a supplicant. I felt defensive and on guard. "I'm not going to go through another medical exam," I muttered to the woman who interviewed me.

I then began the long process of acquiring disability status, which included an examination by a psychiatrist in Cambridge. I was outraged at the suggestion but was told my payments were contingent on passing that hurdle. It was only the first of a long string of humiliations. I sat in his waiting room, fuming inside, surrounded by people who suffered from on-the-job injuries in construction and related areas. When the psychiatrist opened the door and held out his hand, I squeezed it hard enough to hurt, saying, "You look young enough to be my son." He ignored my rudeness and began scribbling some notes on scraps of paper as we talked. After the interview, I asked him why I had to go through this when I was mentally competent. "If you didn't, you wouldn't get your disability. This is supposed to help you." I was immediately ashamed. I now realize he might have been very busy screening out fraudulent claims. Eventually, I did make it through all the hoops put up by Social Security.

To my surprise I also was required to schedule a visit by two staff members of the insurance company, to be followed by an appointment with a urologist the company selected. By that time I felt as if I was continually on the defensive, that everyone doubted I was really ill and was ready to prove it. My husband offered to be present during the home visit and even brought a chair into the living room that was higher than the couch, suggesting I sit there to gain a little advantage. Several of my friends advised me on how to conduct myself during that visit, and one of them who used to administer a nursing home suggested that the company might turn me down even though I had paid for the insurance.

As it turned out, I didn't have to assume a persona. I was myself, weeping with rage and frustration and telling the examiners I would much rather be at work than sitting in the living room with the two of them. The tears upset them and they left immediately, though the presence of my six-foot-two spouse in his business suit sitting next to me may also have hastened their exit.

The final hurdle was a visit to the urologist even though the insurance company had all the medical records from the doctor who had performed my biopsy. My husband and I waited for two and half hours to see the urologist. By the time he called us into his office, I was edgy with fatigue and frustration. The doctor barely listened and didn't take any notes.

Six weeks passed and the urologist still hadn't sent a report to the insurance company. By that time I was experiencing a combination of anger and defeat. Fortunately the anger won out, and I told the claims adjustor I wouldn't be subjected to such a humiliation again; he would have to believe the records or contact the person who had diagnosed me. I was not going to see yet another urologist.

Meanwhile my husband was wrestling with a decision to radically change his career as a manager in a large corporation. Although he enjoyed a number of fringe benefits, he felt increasingly frustrated and stifled in his position. He had received a call from a young man who was in the process of creating a new company and was looking for someone with my husband's skills. It would mean low pay and very long hours, but my husband was more than ready for a new challenge, and he accepted. Mornings, he would drive to Brookline to a small room that served as company headquarters and was also part of a physician's office. It was the beginning of a new and exciting career for him.

I was granted another year at the Wellesley College Center for Research on Women, although my fatigue limited me to a very few of the seminars and events. To an outside observer it might have seemed that I was accomplishing very little, but I was adjusting to a new Marguerite

Bouvard, discovering who she was, what it meant to be ill, and how to help myself. Late one sleepless night I reflected that two of the most profound experiences of my life were taking place simultaneously. One was my illness, which represented one of the most difficult losses that anyone can face, the loss of my very identity, and one of the most difficult fears, that of the unknown. The other experience was my work on the Mothers. I had never struggled so much with a book as I was struggling with this one, because of the immensity of the project and my concern that I couldn't translate my passion into my writing. I wondered how I could create a new self instead of being overcome by my situation.

5

MAP MAKING

I F   I   H A D   heart disease, I thought to myself, I could go to a cardiologist. There were treatments for known illnesses, but not for IC. An empty road stretched out in front of me. I didn't know where to turn for medical care, or how to cope with feeling like a foreigner in my own world. I didn't know how to make it through the day or how to deal with my raging emotions.

I turned to my writing for relief. I lived in my journals, writing in the middle of the night, for now my nights were constantly interrupted. I wrote hunched over the kitchen table in the early hours of the morning. I tucked notebooks in the drawer of my night table and kept them in my study. Even when my mind seemed wrapped in cotton wool, I poured out all my perplexity, filling folder after folder. It was a way of screaming in silence, of letting my pain and rage stamp around in all their fullness. It was also a way of marking time in what seemed like a timeless state.

My nights had become an important part of my history, an underwater world I carried with me. Sitting in the kitchen over a cup of warm milk that I hoped would make me drowsy, I became attuned to sounds that are an undertone throughout the day: the low throb of a refrigerator, the buzz of fluorescent lights, the distant hum of traffic on the highway a block and a half up the hill from our house. I felt as if I were stranded in the middle of an ocean while a world away, on shore, people were sleeping peacefully, gathering strength to enter a day filled with activity.

How could I explain this silent and invisible life to friends and former colleagues? My nocturnal life became a given for me until I traveled. Then the ache of the differences that set me apart from others surfaced.

I was still able to travel to an artists' retreat once a year but found only two that could accommodate my special needs: the Virginia Center for the Creative Arts and, while I could still travel long distances, the Banff Centre for the Performing Arts. When I first applied for and received a residency at Banff in 1991, the administrator not only honored my requests for a special meal; she placed a mattress in my studio so I could rest during the day. I felt fortunate to be among other people again after my long months of working at home in solitude. But mornings, I watched the other artists at the breakfast table with envy. They would call out to me, "Hi Marguerite, come and join us. We were just having a discussion about the new exhibit at the museum in Calgary." My fellow residents were fresh and rested after a good night of sleep and enjoying these moments before the long day of work in their studios. One of the artists was dressed to the nines, sporting a cigarette in a long holder to begin the day, telling jokes and holding court. I had been up so many times the previous night that I was exhausted. I felt as invisible as a mountain peak swathed in cloud. The other artists had no frame of reference for what I was experiencing, so I remained silent.

One day in my studio I reflected that being ill is living on the edge and that I constantly confronted my mortality, my limits. Release would mean I could do the simplest thing without a monumental effort of will and spirit. I could go to bed secure in the expectation of sleep and rest. I wished I had a day to squander mindlessly, believing I was free, encountering people who suffered without really understanding them with my whole being. I felt like someone who had been the unwilling recipient of a terrible tale, or who had stood in the middle of a crowded street caught in mortar fire. (I felt as if I were in Kosovo while the people around me— walking down the street, working at their jobs, or simply having a good time—seemed like vacationers on the Riviera.)

But strangely enough, during these dark times, insights came unexpectedly flooding in, a pattern that would be repeated again and again. One evening during my stay I was lying awake as usual wondering how I could manage the night when a very powerful image came to me. Suddenly my mother was walking ahead of me in a mountain landscape, a landscape so immense I was uncomfortable, but my mother kept walking steadily and I kept following her. That is what generations mean, I concluded—those who have gone before showing us the way, reminding us that we are not the first or the last to have suffered. I remembered my mother recovering on the couch in our living room after she had had a massive heart attack while visiting us, and I felt the chain of being in my guts, not in my head. I remembered how she sewed a beautiful wardrobe for my daughter's doll while she was supposedly resting. I also recalled her decision to fly back to New York before she should have because she wanted her life back.

My mother continued working during her long recovery from the heart attack, when she had to sleep sitting up because she had water in her lungs. She not only kept her job by working out of her apartment but also periodically went to the opera and even visited us to spend time with her grandchildren. The day she died of yet another heart attack, her work-table was filled with sketches, for she was designing a new line for the company where she was both marketing director and dress designer. I had always admired her courage when I was young, watching her deal with a male-oriented world at work and struggling to make ends meet as a single mother. In contrast to my father's intermittent and often difficult presence in my life, she was loving and consistent. Even though she had died twenty years ago, I realized that she was still with me, guiding me through life by her example and her unfailing support.

Despite the differences that set me apart from others, the weeks I was able to spend at such retreats were a privilege. They helped me to feel like a part of a working world again rather than like someone living on the margins. Throughout my stays there were always opportunities to attend readings of work in progress, art exhibits, and music performances of the resident artists. There was the happiness of long conversations about each other's work over dinner in the cafeteria and occasional walks with one of the artists.

I remembered how I had previously ended my stays in such places with reluctance, feeling that I would have too little time to write given my hectic life and crowded teaching schedule. Now I felt reluctant to return home, where I would work alone and without a schedule.

While I was floundering in my new condition, my husband was also at a loss. He wanted to help but didn't know quite what to do. I didn't know either how to ask for help or what kind of help I needed. At the time, my husband had a punishing working schedule, and I didn't wish to become a burden. Once, after a very difficult night, I saw him beaming in my study. He had organized my poetry books alphabetically and transferred the titles to my computer. I was deeply touched.

๛๛๛

What held me together during this period was not only my brief forays to writers' retreats but also my book about the Mothers of the Plaza de

Mayo. There was a parallel between my efforts to write about the Mothers and my attempts to reorient myself in the world of the ill. I had no guidelines for either endeavor. For the very first time, I was working on a book without a set of concepts or a theoretical framework. Deciding how to tell the Mothers' story, I felt like a detective gathering pieces of a puzzle. There were no historical precedents for a national movement founded by elderly women most of whom had once lived in quiet domesticity and, with a few exceptions, rarely read a newspaper. In the midst of state terrorism, a group of mothers had formed a collective based on direct democracy and ties of affection, a group of women who offended most middle-class feminists in Latin America and the United States by their seeming lack of organization and their radical politics.

I traced their political style to the anarchist movement in Spain during the Civil War, when peaceful cooperatives sprang up spontaneously as a source of order in a turbulent world. I had studied Spanish anarchism as a graduate student, and one of the Mothers, Mercedes Mereño, had emigrated from Spain during that war because her father was shot before her eyes for his work as a labor union leader. She brought with her a respect for the power of spontaneous grassroots movements unattached to any political parties.

While pondering my approach I read Sara Ruddick's *Maternal Thinking*, a revelation because it not only helped me understand the Mothers but also affirmed my own experience that feelings are central to living well. When I was preparing for my doctorate in the 1960s, "objectivity" was defined by a male-dominated culture as not only a lack of bias but also a perspective free of emotion, implying that feelings are both dangerous and lacking intelligence. Nor was there any attempt in this wholesale dismissal of the emotions to distinguish between those that can harm others, such as hatred, and those that are important in living fully. If ignoring the wisdom of affect was part of academic life, I found its absence blatant in the world of the ill and in the way women activists were viewed. In Argentina, the bias against expressing feelings enabled the government to dismiss the Mothers as hysterical women.

It was the Mothers and not academic thinkers who revealed the political usefulness and the power of informed emotion. Expressing their grief and anger publicly in their demonstrations not only broke a cultural taboo but also enhanced their political effectiveness. This was the first time women rose up to organize and lead resistance in a way that reflected maternal values. It took me some time before I was able to give myself permission to write their story using both my emotional and my intellectual resources.

I saw much of my own life nested in the Mothers' story, where the private and public were intermingled in new ways, especially in their way of organizing their work. Multitasking is a talent that flourishes in the private sphere and that has always served women well. Although there was now a yawning gap between my private and my public life, I was learning in a new way to draw on the strengths of my previous experiences of bringing up my children and of volunteering as well as those I developed in my long months at home. These experiences enabled me to write the Mothers' story in a way that would encompass the totality of their accomplishments as women, not just their political efforts.

While writing, I focused on the Mothers' chaotic days at their office, punctuated by their forays into the streets and responses to threatening phone calls or to people who came in for help at all hours. I too lived in chaos, for each day was different, depending on the quality of my nights and how I felt. I usually managed at least a half hour at my desk, but it could be in the morning, afternoon, or night. I also spent time on the telephone, reading, and listening to my collection of classical music. I found myself negotiating each moment, for I had to run to the bathroom frequently, and that plus my fatigue kept me homebound much of the time. I lost the spontaneity I had once taken for granted, but in a strange way I experienced a continuity in my work, for listening to music, or even reading my collection of art history books, was not only a respite but also a way of thinking about the problems I was having with my book. I too learned how I could work toward my goals in an unpredictable fashion.

My vision as a poet helped me navigate my illness and create a way of understanding the Mothers, for there are no taboo subjects in poetry; like so many before me, I could write poems about living with my situation. Poetry breaks the silence of social correctness and invades all the spaces of the politically powerful, causing many oppressive governments around the world to exile or imprison writers. The Mothers invaded the privileged space of governmental discourse by forming their own language and proclaiming it publicly. When the newly elected president Raul Alfonsin took power, he kept repeating the need to heal the wounds of the nation. The Mothers responded with "Let there be no healing of wounds. Because if the wounds still bleed there will be no forgetting." The Mothers used the space of the streets and plazas in a society where woman are supposed to remain at home. They began to publish their own newspaper, books, and pamphlets when they were denied coverage in the national press. They were everywhere, continually oozing through and around established structures in order to be heard and to remain visible. As the years passed, I would see the Mothers before me when I would work to find a public role for myself over and beyond my writing by giving presentations on aspects of chronic illness.

Over four years of writing and reflecting I created a new framework out of disparate pieces, and was able to complete the book in 1994. An Italian astrophysicist I watched on a television program claimed that the laws of physics did not apply to black holes, that we would have to invent an entirely new science to define that phenomenon. Without realizing it, I was gathering the fragments of my life and reassembling them into my own new physics to define a way for myself as well as understanding the enormity of what the Mothers had achieved. When I first set out for Argentina in 1989, I never thought that my experience with the Mothers would both mirror the new reality of my illness and help me rebuild my life. My passion for this project would hold me together, ferrying me through such trying circumstances.

꙳꙳꙳

I was leading a double life, one part devoted to my work as a writer, the other filled with the hard and invisible work of finding appropriate medical care, an ongoing project. In fact, it took me many years to think of this attempt to manage my illness as part of my work. In 1991, while I was immersed in the book, the body I once blithely ignored demanded my continual attention. Whenever I was out or driving somewhere I worried about finding a bathroom, for urinary frequency is a continual problem I face. At first I didn't even think of trying to research IC but looked for ways of alleviating my symptoms, only to find that there were no proven treatments aside from the anti-inflammatory DMSO instillations, which didn't help me. I was suddenly in charge of my health even though I had no medical knowledge.

I gave up consulting urologists when I asked the specialist I was seeing if I could get Elmiron on "compassionate use," a drug I learned about from other women with IC who were taking it with success (physicians often resort to compassionate use to obtain a drug for patients in distress before FDA approval). At first he assented, but when my husband left a meeting to finalize the papers for such a request, the physician came into the consulting room holding my file and not even looking at us. He sat down, still without making eye contact, and said, "I no longer recommend this treatment. Besides, women with IC are prone to commit suicide, and divorces often result from the toll of this illness." My husband and I remained speechless with surprise. Later we both wrote a letter of complaint. Those words sunk into my flesh, and I vowed to stay away from urologists.

Instead I decided to try alternative medicine, turning to the fringes of Eastern techniques, Reiki in particular. The alternative clinic I attended in Watertown in 1991 made me feel as if I were back in the 1960s. Its many slightly seedy rooms, which once served as classrooms, were buzzing with activity and with bearded young men wearing earnest expressions. Sounds of New Age music wafted through the halls, soft, soothing, but a cut above Muzak. I remembered a book I had written about communes many years ago. Now I felt that I had returned to that period, when living in community with little regard for such antediluvian customs as personal clothing, marriage, and privacy was supposed to cure all social ills. I was ushered into a darkened room where a so-called healer held his hands above my bladder and went into meditation.

"You will feel a warmth just above your bladder," Steve whispered, holding his hands above my bladder. I still don't know whether it was the power of suggestion, but I did feel that warmth and slept better that night. In my enthusiasm I asked to see him once a week, instead of the intermittent schedule he had available. He assented readily and suggested I go to his home in Cambridge.

The following Thursday I was climbing the stairs to the second floor of his home, noticing with disgust the piles of papers and soiled clothes abandoned throughout the rooms. The room where he "healed" was not as cluttered as the others, and we went into meditation accompanied by the soft whisper of distant gongs and cymbals.

When the hour was up, he told me in a very businesslike tone of voice that I owed him seventy-five dollars. I wrote out the check and fled. It was the end of Reiki as far as I was concerned. I had fallen with eyes wide open into what my husband called an *attrape nigaud*, loosely translated as a lure for fools.

I then attended a mind-body clinic at the Deaconess Hospital for a six-week course on meditation. The director was warm and welcoming. She inspired confidence, since she had written a number of excellent books and studied in India for many years. It was the first time I was in a room with so many other ill people.

We were learning how to meditate. I had been meditating for some time before this but not very seriously. In the mid-1980s, a friend from my women's network told me about learning how to meditate. It seemed that everyone was meditating those days: TM, it was called, for transcendental meditation. I asked her how and where she learned, and she told me about the Self-Realization Fellowship in Encinitas, California, that she had joined. I was of two minds, wondering whether this was just another California "trip" or something serious. I read a book she suggested, *Autobiography of a Yoga*, by Parmahansa Yogananda, and decided to write to the center he had founded in Encinitas. Because I was so busy, I sent away for lessons and received thirty-eight over a period of several months.

This was new territory for me. I learned to repeat *om* to myself, to focus. At first I could sit only for five minutes, and even that seemed an eternity. Eventually I completed the lessons, working my way up to ten minutes, a practice that also took an effort. Every morning before leaving for work I meditated for ten minutes, hoping to relieve the stress of my working situation. I believed I was meditating, but I hadn't really learned. It was only in the third year of illness that my meditation deepened and I began to truly focus. It was no longer about work-related stress but about the loneliness of living with so many physical constraints and the realization of the extent of my loss.

At the Deaconess Hospital we were learning to use the mind on behalf of the body as some twenty of us were seated on the floor in a dimly lit room. I was not quite ready for this, because I still didn't understand the nature or prognosis of this illness, but it was a comfort to be among others who were in similar situations. There was a cardiologist among us who wanted to help his patients and also a high-powered businessman who attended the sessions because he wanted to reduce the stress in his life. As we went into meditation, he usually responded by falling asleep and snoring loudly. I chuckled at the absurdity of our lives.

I also looked for a support group, but while cancer recovery groups were abundant, I had difficulty finding a group for the chronically ill. I called a center that sponsors cancer support groups unaffiliated to a hospital, and the director informed me that there were none for chronic illnesses. After a year's searching, the same center sent me a brochure about a support group that seemed to fit my needs.

In the fall of 1992, I sat among a group of people recounting stories of difficulties in getting diagnoses, unfeeling responses from doctors, and the ache of being thrust into unfathomable situations. One young woman shared a conversation with a physician in which he asked her, "Are you married?" When she replied that she wasn't, he retorted, "Well you want to be!" We all laughed in recognition of similar conversations.

But while there were light moments, I discovered that the boundaries I once had, however thin, were gone and that everyone's emotional pain seeped into my pores. While such an alternative is useful for many people, I turned to one of the group leaders, a social worker, for one-on-one support.

She not only taught me how to speak with doctors but also introduced me to the world of East-West medicine, which proved helpful in easing pain and fatigue. I entered the strange country of vitamins, herbal remedies, homeopathy, and reflexology. What seemed most important about these approaches was the dialogue with the practitioner. Even though IC affects the immune system of some people who suffer from it, none of the specialists I had consulted believed my stories of fatigue. But the holistic doctor I began seeing, Dr. Glen Rothfeld, considered me in my entirety. He immediately discovered I had vitamin and mineral deficiencies from the fatigue that was plaguing me, and I began taking weekly intravenous injections to strengthen my body. When that proved no longer helpful, I tried acupuncture to relax me and relieve the pain. The practitioners talked to me as they inserted the needles: I could discuss my illness without feeling I had to keep quiet and assume a cheerful demeanor.

When the acupuncturist in this practice moved to another state, I was put in touch with a most delightful and eccentric acupuncturist from China who had a prickly exterior and a very warm heart. She also became an important role model, for after I had seen her a number of times, she told me about her imprisonment during the Cultural Revolution in China, when she had considered taking her own life because the conditions were so terrible; about her neurologist husband, who had abandoned her; and about the barriers to achieving recognition from the medical establishments in the Boston area. "It is difficult to be a woman; it is even more difficult to be a Chinese woman," she once commented to me. Listening to her stories about her trials and witnessing her bravery and ingenuity in carving out a life for herself became as important as the treatments.

Her daughter was then a medical student who "makes As while other students who do not have to learn English make Cs." We discussed our concerns about and our pride in our daughters at great length. We were mothers, not only doctor and patient. Because of this, I felt that I was in a position of sharing and equality, a satisfying relationship, unlike that of the authoritative physician and the compliant patient.

Dr. Chen did everything she could for me, even trying the ancient practice of cupping one afternoon (placing heated cups on the body to stimulate circulation). One day when I was feeling particularly ill she told me, "You stay here, I'll be back soon," and stepped out of her office while I lay there with the needles wobbling on me. About a half hour later, she returned with some of her homemade chicken soup. "Italian penicillin," my mother used to call it, but it's also Chinese and Jewish penicillin. She even tried heat lamps she had brought back from China during one of her yearly trips. To boost my energy, she sold me herbal medicine that she reserved for her cancer patients, and she always kept my spirits up.

I reluctantly terminated my visits when I no longer experienced an alleviation of pain.

᠊ᢌᢌᢌ᠊

It was by sheer accident that I was put in touch with a new urologist who treated me with respect and caring. I was having a gynecological visit in my HMO in 1992, because gynecological problems are a part of IC, when the doctor told me his nurse had IC and suggested we talk to each other. She told me about the urologist she had been consulting in St. Elizabeth's hospital in Brighton, and I felt hopeful.

It took months to get an appointment, but when I saw this young woman's physician I was pleasantly surprised. Dr. Pais was gentle and courteous, and discussed diet with me. He decided to perform a cystoscopy in order to examine the condition of my bladder, removing a polyp. Even though my insurance didn't allow overnight stays in the hospital, he was kind enough to tell them that he needed to have me under observation just so I could recover.

I scheduled another visit to try an instillation of the anti-inflammatory DMSO again when his younger partner, Dr. Coukos, asked me to step into his office simply because he wanted to talk about my case. By now, I was amazed to be so well treated and felt very grateful. After almost five years, I had finally found a specialist who was willing to work with me, took a genuine interest in me, and never called me by my first name.

Meanwhile I started reading up on IC. The national Interstitial Cystitis Association,[1] which I joined, sends out quarterly bulletins with abstracts

1. The ICA is a national organization that funds research on IC, educates the medical community and the public, and supports patients with counseling, referrals, and information about interstitial cystitis.

of medical articles and discussions with doctors about this condition. It also sells articles that have served as guides in dealing with IC. I am grateful, for it responds to the myriad aspects of this perplexing disease and speaks to the fact the majority of sufferers are women. It is headed by Dr. Vicki Ratner, a urologist who also has IC, and who founded the organization as a nationwide network for fund-raising to support research on this baffling illness.

When I speak to women from around the country twice a year for the purpose of fund-raising for the national Interstitial Cystitis Organization, we spend considerable time discussing our situations. It makes me feel less crazy when I hear from other women about similar symptoms that doctors find puzzling and unaccountable. I was relieved that I was not the only person to find that department stores exacerbate my fatigue and make me feel nauseated. I learned that this is caused by the heavy presence of perfume and, since then, have stopped wearing anything scented and avoid shopping. I felt less alone when I spoke with a woman who told me that she couldn't tolerate more than twenty minutes in the car and that she too battled fatigue. We compared treatments and symptoms.

These conversations and the articles I culled from the newsletter and the World Wide Web helped me along the road to taking charge of my own care, for it was not and is still not possible to find a primary care physician who has sufficient time, resources, and knowledge about IC, and there are very few urologists who know much about this illness.

In the fall of 1992, I found an article in the *Interstitial Cystitis Quarterly Newsletter* about a new treatment called Cystistat or hyaluronic acid, a highly refined product made from the connective tissue of rooster combs. Cystistat temporarily replaces the gag layer of the bladder, which is typically damaged and inflamed in IC sufferers. The gag layer is the glycosaminoglycan layer, or hyaluronate, that people naturally produce on the bladder epithelium and that is believed to provide a protective coating on the bladder wall. Cystistat is supposed to have effects similar to those of Elmiron (pentosan polysulfate sodium), a medication that became available in 1998, although by then many women were already taking it. I immediately researched this medicine and discovered that it was produced in a small laboratory in Toronto, Canada, but unavailable in the United States because there had been no studies on Cystistat and therefore doctors were not authorized by the FDA to use it.

However, one year later, in 1993, I discovered that a handful of doctors were using it in Colorado and Illinois. Yet another year passed until the FDA authorized its use by urologists around the country. Dr. Coukos agreed to let me try it, and in 1994 I began importing Cystistat periodically from Canada for monthly instillations. After so many years without an alleviation of my symptoms, it was the first medication that worked for me. I felt most fortunate because it provides relief for only about 45 percent of IC patients.

At the same time I saw an article in the IC newsletter about the availability of a card identifying a person as an IC patient with problems of urgency. I immediately sent away for one, and it has proved invaluable in getting me to the head of the line that always gathers before public women's rooms. Finding a bathroom is always uppermost on my mind whenever I go out, but standing in line is also an issue. Such details of everyday life, which I had rarely thought about before, had become part and parcel of finding appropriate medical care.

꒰ ꒰ ꒰

In tandem with reading about IC, I also read voraciously about illness in general, most particularly books by contemporary doctors and writers who promised instant healing, perfect health, and long life. Browsing through Waterstone's in Boston one morning, I was struck by the number of books on health and the mind. In a society that worships health, it seemed an affront to be ill. I had not only fallen ill; I failed to get well rapidly. Such an attitude is reminiscent of contemporary views of the poor, as if somehow the healthy and the well were exempted from suffering on account of their inherent superiority.

But then I was directed to Steven Levine's *Healing into Life and Death*. His meditation techniques, his suggestions on "sitting with pain," his explorations of illness by reconnecting the mind/body/heart were deeply comforting and led me down a new path. During meditation, I shut my study door for privacy and confronted myself, often letting the tears roll down my cheeks. It helped me to face and honor my discouragement and pain, to feel "how will I ever get through this?" It was a place to bring my sorrow and grief. Ultimately it helped me overcome my acute sense of loss until it became a strand in my days, off center, not a boulder crushing my chest.

I read books on spirituality as well, for serious illness has a way of thrusting a person headlong into his or her inner space. For me, it was like a jolt awakening me to a deeper reality where the issues I faced centered on survival and how to continue living well, rather than the more mundane problems of my previous life. I found myself grappling not only with meaning but also with a new desire to explore this inner space. Although I have always been deeply religious, and although I had been brought up Catholic, from early childhood I rebelled against the church's strictures: I feel more comfortable combining a variety of religious outlooks. I turned to *The Practice of the Presence of God*, written in the mid-1600s by Brother Lawrence of the Resurrection; Thomas Moore's *Care of the Soul*; and the Buddhist writer Sharon Salzberg's *Heart as Wide as the World*. I have always been interested in Zen Buddhism and, thanks to my daughter, have a large collection of books on that topic. I even read the Buddhist bible and Rebbe Nachman of Breslov, the Hasidic mystic whose life spanned the eighteenth and nineteenth centuries. What these books had in common was the revelation of how the ordinary events of our everyday lives are suffused with spirituality, how every moment we have is somehow extraordinary in its own way. Rebbe Nachman's writings opened me up in a new way to the immensity and the mystery that surrounds us, and how our brief flickers are part of a much larger order. I came to feel our profound connectedness with my whole being, and it brought a feeling of spaciousness to my seemingly cramped days.

Inspired by my friend Awiakta and by my time at the conference on women and leadership, I began studying Native American history and poetry and especially the writings of their spiritual leaders. I acquired a new view of the sacredness of nature and hence of the body. Although I had always experienced the wonder of the creation, these explorations helped me place my own problems off center. I learned a new perspective; although I was not able to change my circumstances, I could transform my attitudes.

⚹ ⚹ ⚹

One of the hardest things for me was coordinating my care. It seemed as if each of my body parts was demanding attention and that I was in charge of a refractory group of children. My attention jumped from the pain in my bladder to the pain in my pelvis to the overwhelming fatigue I was experiencing. How they were related was a mystery I couldn't begin to fathom. At the time, all I knew was that my whole body was crying out while I went from one specialist to another, feeling that I was being reduced to a modular creature. My female organs were entrusted to a gynecologist, my bladder to a urologist; and my difficulty sleeping had already led me to consult a psychopharmacologist.

While I was at the retreat in Banff in 1992, one of the writers gave me one of her Valium tablets to help ease my night. It did make a difference, and the following year I went to consult a psychopharmacologist to help me with sleep as well as with pain. He prescribed Klonopin, an anti-seizure medication (with IC, bladders frequently go into spasm) and a tranquilizer. Pain is a problem I have had to live with, for I found that I am allergic to most painkillers and to the antidepressants such as Elevil and Norpramin commonly given IC patients to alleviate their distress. Even such a simple over-the-counter remedy as Advil has side effects I am unable to tolerate. But strangely enough, after years of acting as a combatant I suddenly and unconsciously surrendered to pain. I learned not to tense when it invades me but rather to relax and just notice it as if it were happening to someone else. Pain is no longer exotic but familiar, and I am even able to sleep while being aware of it. That discovery came out of my practice of meditation, helping me to accept the new terms of my life.

I also learned that exercise is supposed to help the immune system, and when the winter snows melt I try (but can't always manage) to take walks twice a week. They do give me a spurt of energy. Swimming in a pool is not an option, because the chlorine causes pain. Treadmills are also particularly hard on many of us with IC, but walking is a wonderful sport, refreshing my spirit as well as my body. I am lucky to live near a trail that borders a lake where I can mark the changing of the seasons and admire the trees. However, like many women who have IC, I have had to learn to live with relentless exhaustion.

It is very difficult to discuss this fatigue with most physicians. All too often our conversations are technical and could be about areas in a construction site rather than about my own flesh, the wholeness of me. My monthly visits for Cystistat instillations were the exception. The young woman who performed these procedures for the first five years, Lisa Cautillo, was a physician's assistant. She always took extra time with me, knowing about my sensitivity to pain, and she always inquired how I was feeling. Often, while I was lying down on the examining table before she began, she sat by my side to chat. It may seem like a small gesture, but the arrangement of space between doctor and patient, with the physician towering over my body, makes me feel diminished.

Because IC is frequently accompanied by gynecological problems such as vulvodynia, a condition of vulvar pain, I began to think about hormone replacement, which is supposed to help such conditions. A friend put me touch with the head of the Vincent Memorial Obstetrics and Gynecology Services at the Massachusetts General Hospital. Dr. Schiff exuded the dignity of the highly competent, expressing genuine concern. We discussed my age and the risks at great length. I was not a cipher for him or another file. When the progesterone that is taken to counteract the risk of cancer worsened my IC symptoms, he agreed to supervise me with a very low dose of local estrogen cream provided I check in with him regularly and have a yearly biopsy and half-yearly ultrasound. Making this decision assuaged the feeling of powerlessness that often overwhelms me and that accompanies chronic illness.

In fact, whenever I have a consultation with Dr. Schiff, he shows me my file and we peruse it together. I feel that we are in a partnership and that he values my insights. My various experiences with some of my doctors as well as my efforts to create a new life have altered my perceptions of healing. The physicians who have helped me the most have done so primarily because they recognized me as a whole person and because of their empathy. People with disabilities want to be treated with respect and to have the complete range of their symptoms acknowledged as well as the fact that they have full lives.

In his book *The Wounded Storyteller*, Arthur Frank reveals the extent to which doctors have taken over both the language and the experience of illness. He refers to illness stories as rescuing our sovereignty over our own lives. As so many ill people have painfully discovered, there is no accepted space or language for the pain, discouragement, and illuminations we experience. Until I had the good fortune to find physicians like Dr. Schiff, I typically was made to feel as if the totality of my life was insignificant.

The Pulitzer Prize–winning play *W;t* by Margaret Edson is a wonderful parody of the yawning gulf between what I would refer to as medi-speak and one woman's experience with terminal cancer. It is a perfect example of what Arthur Frank referred to as "being colonized," having her story of suffering suppressed. During the grand rounds, the fellows surrounding her physicians examine her body. "Then one of the fellows pipes up 'Very late detection staged as a four upon admission. Hexamethophosphacil with vinplatin to potentiate.'"[2] As he continues his lengthy analysis, and as the fellows gape at her body, the woman thinks that the term *rounds* is really running around the main issue, her life, her struggle.

---

2. M. Edson, *W;t* (Faber & Faber, New York, 2000), 36.

I remember a preoperative discussion with an anesthesiologist in which I informed him of the problems I was experiencing with IC. "Other than that you are perfectly healthy?" he inquired. I looked at him scathingly, but he was blithely unaware the effect of his words. Later I imagined how I would have liked to douse him with a glass of water, telling him, "Other than that you are perfectly dry?"

The fact that coping with illness is both rich and significant often seems to elude some physicians. I remember a psychopharmacologist who used to periodically review my medications with me, asking me with genuine perplexity, "What do you do all day?" I gasped and mumbled something about cleaning up my files from my previous books. But when I got home, I sat down and wrote in my journal: *what I do all day: I talk on the telephone to my daughter and rejoice with her when she's had a good job voicing an advertisement. I talk to a friend whose husband is dying slowly and painfully. I read, I write letters, go over my e-mail, sometimes have an hour for my writing, I cook dinner.* The fact that I do not have a schedule, that every single day is different depending on the kind of night I have had and the level of pain I am experiencing, makes it even more difficult to explain exactly how I spend my time. I want to shout out, "It's possible to live the way I do, without predictability and in chaos! It's demanding, exhausting, but I've learned flexibility." Suffering does not mean the absence of life. The heart still beats, still speaks to the world.

❧ ❧ ❧

One of the hardest lessons for me was paying attention to the body I had ignored for so many years. I was never terribly interested in exercise and would work as if I had no limits. Now I listen to my body very carefully: it tells me about stress, about what is happening in my life, and what it may need at the moment. In an age when people in our society are trying to control their bodies by working out, dieting, or having cosmetic surgery, I began to respect mine in a new way. When my enthusiasm too often draws me beyond my limits, I spend many days recovering; but honoring my passions is worth these setbacks. For instance, attending a seminar at a local university on a subject that happens to interest me is important to me even though it may last two hours or more and means I must give up my nap. Such events feed my soul for many weeks and serve as flint for my work.

Among the features of this illness in my case are unpredictable flare-ups during which I go through many weeks of bladder spasms, lack of sleep, and extreme pain that feels as if a knife is scouring my bladder. These often seem like long winter months when I struggle to maintain my sense of self-worth even though the list of things I cannot do seems endless. However, mornings I always dress as if I were going out, a small gesture that helps me to feel I am not giving in to my circumstances. Sometimes I am able to do the detail jobs in support of my writing—making telephone calls, sorting my papers, and filing—tasks that do not take mental concentration. But often I am just resting, doing the invisible work of sickness that is so demanding, not only of the body but also, especially, of the heart and spirit. I think of adventurers like Sir Ernest Shackleton, who voyaged to the Antarctic in 1914, testing himself against the cold, the unpredictability of ice, the soft ice turning to cement or the harder layers slowly closing off the open waters and stranding him for months. In my case, the elements are within myself.

When in the midst of one of these difficult periods, I focus on crossing the terrain of my day, trying not to think of what I would want to do or what others are doing. I concentrate on neither feeling too much nor wasting precious energy on regret. I think of the prisoners described in Solzhenitsyn's *First Circle* who learned to walk very slowly in order to conserve energy because they were placed on a starvation diet as torture and humiliation. Thus they lessened the tyranny of hunger, and thus I lessen the tyranny of my illness.

I also have rare days when I am feeling so well I am euphoric. If I had a voice, I would sing at the top of my lungs; if I were athletic, I would turn cartwheels on our lawn. Sometimes I celebrate by taking a walk by Lake Waban with my husband, watching a flock of gulls settling in the middle of the lake, the patterns of fractured ice, and breathing in the wonderful presence of the woods that border the path. Then I think that people do not understand the true happiness of being alive.

6

HUMAN RIGHTS REVISITED

ALTHOUGH in the early years of my illness I felt as if the life I had so carefully built was over, it was in the depths of a solitude I believed would be a permanent condition that I began the hard work of rewriting my life. I redefined and expanded what I came to consider as the narrow social concepts of work to include the many tasks around illness. I integrated these efforts with trying to remain engaged in the world by creating a new public identity. It proved to be a sometimes overwhelming, multifaceted, and ongoing work, for a life is filled with many different aspects we rarely think about, because they have become routine. I had no more routines. I needed to create ways of living well with unpredictability and to translate my reality into the language of the healthy.

My passion for human rights was still in the forefront of my goals, but now that I had accepted my own situation, I found that passion enlarged. I became increasingly concerned with the social images and the rights of the disabled as well as with creating a discourse that would bridge the worlds of the healthy and the ill. These pursuits would become intertwined as I tried to find a setting where I could carry on my work among colleagues.

My first experience in becoming an advocate for the ill happened spontaneously. In 1993 I flew to Long Beach, California, to give a presentation on coping with grief at a national conference of hospice workers. I arrived with a prepared talk focused on grieving, based on a book I had written. While I was at a social gathering for all the attendees the night before the proceedings would begin, I heard a priest referring to the *"unfortunates who are ill."* Although he and I later became very friendly, that remark sent me speeding back to my hotel room in a rage. I ripped up my speech and began writing a new one.

The following day I spoke not only about allowing oneself to experience the turbulence of emotions around loss as a path to healing but also about my personal experience: "Perhaps one way to create a common social discourse is to think of ourselves as not only defined by our careers or social roles, however necessary these categorizations are, but also as members of a circle of being, held together by a web of common experiences and possibilities. In my struggles as an ill person I discovered that the line between illness and health, good luck and bad is a very thin one. If we recognize ourselves in those who suffer, we can heal ourselves and our society." I gave special emphasis to the intrinsic value of the invisible storms of grief over illness and talked about the importance of anger, not as wrath directed against myself or against others with the intention of causing harm, but as a healthy aggression leading to inner transformation and empowerment. Surprisingly, a number of people came up to me afterward wanting to talk about their own experiences, including a woman who had multiple sclerosis.

After the conference I wrote an article from my presentation for a magazine intended for hospice workers and the clergy, and soon found myself writing more pieces about living with illness. I felt a need to awaken people to a reality so different from their own even though they were caregivers. But some years would pass before I would begin to approach the need for discourse in a more intense and systematic way. Since that conference many books have appeared on bereavement, yet there has been little public acknowledgment of the tremendous, invisible work of coping with chronic conditions.

For me, part of that work is adjusting to the daily changes in how I am feeling and to my moments of comparing myself with other people who seem to swim through the day like dolphins. Chronic illness has its own calendar and rhythms. It takes place outside the normal sequence of periods of work and rest, of days unfolding in a predictable manner. My mornings, afternoons, and evenings are tangled, and often my nights are wakeful substitutes for days. No single day resembles another. I may have weeks when I am feeling well enough to work for a few hours at different times of the day or night followed by weeks where I must rest.

꙳ ꙳ ꙳

In 1992 someone I knew who was in residence at Brandeis University suggested that I apply to the Women's Studies Program as a visiting scholar. I was still mourning my former life at the college, wishing I could be in the classroom again, a professor, not an ill person. I was also nervous about applying because of my battered self-esteem. I kept putting it off, but and my friend kept urging me on with her charming Brooklyn accent, "Just caul Marguerite, caul." I finally mustered the courage to contact the director of the program, Shulamit Reinharz. To my surprise, Shula was both warm and welcoming, suggesting I send her a letter with my résumé as well as ideas about what I might do for the program. She invited me to lunch before the end of our conversation. Reentering academic society no longer seemed like an insuperable effort.

A week later we met, and a door opened to a new life. Shula certainly didn't fit my vision of an academic program director. She looked more like a svelte athlete, exuding energy and especially practicality. We had a wonderful discussion about our interests, and then she asked me, "What would you like to do here?" implying that I would have free rein as well as financial support for my projects. Coming from a college where I had had little or no support for programs to enrich my courses, I could hardly absorb this. I told her about my interest in human rights and that I would like to establish a lecture series on women and human rights. Fine, Shula answered. "I think it would be a good idea for you to attend the next meeting of the board of trustees for the program and make a presentation about your project."

I had never attended a meeting of all-women trustees, especially a group so eager to lend their support for women's studies. A woman with masses of light, curly hair, who radiated warmth, came up to me after my presentation proposing the lecture series. She patted me on the arm and assured me, "You'll have the funds you need." I later discovered that she was a noted philanthropist who had lived through repeated bouts of cancer.

I came home in a cloud of happiness. Because of my former activism I had a long list of contacts, and preparing such a program was something I could accomplish with telephone calls. Brandeis didn't have electronic mail then, but Shula and I made frequent use of the fax machine and soon the first lecture was in place. Once I had made the arrangements, and had discussed the publicity and the flyers with the coordinator of the program, all I needed to do was to introduce the speakers and field questions for them. Suddenly staying at home all day no longer seemed so confining.

The series opened that autumn with an inspiring presentation by Vera Laska, who had spent years in the Resistance against the Nazi occupation of Czechoslovakia while only a teenager. The auditorium was packed, and it throbbed with excitement. Over seventy-five people attended, and after Vera's talk the questions came pouring in thick and fast. I felt as if I were in the classroom again. Vera's experiences resonated; I was certain that the audience would walk away transformed. I also experienced joy at finding a new way of participating in a world that meant so much to me.

At my former college, I used to arrange for guest speakers as a matter of course, chauffeuring them about and taking them to dinner to compensate for the low honoraria. It was one thread in my very crowded days of teaching. After this experience at Brandeis, I learned that I could feel just as fulfilled, perhaps even more so, by accomplishing one thing. I learned that what I do rather than how much is what matters.

The program was such a success that I decided to try bringing the Mothers of the Plaza de Mayo to the United States. Although they had frequently traveled to contact members of the U.S. Senate and government officials in the early years of their political efforts, they refused to return when President Ronald Reagan, replacing President Jimmy Carter, resumed trade with the military junta, a policy continued by President George Bush.

After two years with the Women's Studies Scholars Program I knew that I would find support to bring one Mother over. I discussed this with Shula and as usual she was very responsive, suggesting that I once again join the annual meeting of the board of directors of the program to present my proposal. Happily the project received a major grant for the program to hold yearly symposia, so that two of the Mothers were able to fly to Boston in 1994.

I had free rein to design the symposium, and I worked long and hard but at my own pace, on my own chaotic schedule. I planned to share this event with as many people as possible and to make it a complete experience, with a play about the Mothers the evening prior to their presentation and a discussion with a panel of noted scholars. I contacted Lavonne Mueller, whose moving play about the Mothers' story had been produced in London, and she agreed to let us use the script. A member of the Theater Department at Brandeis, Susan Dibble, offered to direct the reading of the play, and the department provided the cast.

After a year of faxing, telephoning, and scheduling meetings, combined with my strange life of naps, interrupted nights, and doctors' appointments, the Mothers' weekend became a reality. My whole family joined in. My son Pierre flew in from New York City to drive the Mothers to their various interviews on television and radio; I wanted the Mothers to get as much publicity as possible during this trip. My actress daughter traveled from London to take part in the production, and my husband took the day off to pick up the Mothers at the airport.

It seemed like a dream when Juana de Pargament and Mercedes Mereño walked into the crowded waiting room of the airport and we embraced. They had had a long and punishing trip, but as usual they were full of plans and enthusiasm. "There is so much to do," Juana told me. "The Mothers must go to Korea and speak to the mothers there, and then there are the problems in the Middle East."

When we arrived at our home and after I served them tea, Juana and Mercedes immediately began their preparations for the next day. They stayed with us because I wanted them to be comfortable and because they didn't speak English. Between my daughter Laurence's fluent Italian and my stumbling Spanish we managed beautifully.

But the next morning I received a strange phone call from a man speaking in a thick Argentine accent; then he hung up before I could respond. I immediately contacted Shula, and she provided security guards at the university to ensure the Mothers' safety.

The symposium began on Friday night with a reading of the play, and I was touched to see some of my former colleagues in the audience. On Saturday there was a lunch for the Mothers before a panel of scholars I organized and in which I participated. While we were eating, the doors were locked and the security guards stood outside the room. But when the Mothers walked into the auditorium, hundreds of students and people from surrounding communities as well as journalists began clapping and cheering. Shula read out telegrams of congratulations from local politicians as well as from notable human rights activists. The campus was electric with excitement.

Shula provided a room for me on campus where I could rest, but although I lay down, I was too wound up to sleep. I was swept by my utter joy at being with the Mothers again and the fortuitous publication of my book about them. I was too tired to attend the evening festivities, which included a movie about the Mothers featuring the noted actress Liv Ullmann, but that didn't matter. I had made it through the day. The following morning I was still asleep when my husband drove the Mothers to the airport, but they understood and were busy preparing for their coming appearances in New York City.

☙☙☙

Those first two years, there were only a few scholars in the program: two and then four. But the Women's Studies Scholars Program very quickly drew applicants from highly talented women in many different fields until today it is a vibrant community of over sixty scholars. Among them are a composer, a neurotoxicologist, a public defender and writer, an investigative journalist, a biologist, a cultural anthropologist, a former secretary of state of economic affairs in Massachusetts concerned with women's wages, a filmmaker, as well as a conductor and manager of a woman's chorus, a cellist—in short a highly diverse group. Many of these women are simultaneously pursuing two careers, including one scholar who recently became a sculptress subsequent to teaching and working in academic administration.

Not surprisingly, many scholars are political activists in addition to their writing and research. For example, one writer is supporting the construction of a high school in Nicaragua, another works on behalf of poor Latina women in the Boston area, and the community as a whole often participates in one woman's efforts on behalf of a cause such as supporting young women recently rescued from sexual slavery.

The importance of political activism among other scholars, as well as being with women artists, scholars, and professionals who had worked outside socially established boundaries, made me feel as if I had come home. At my former college, the fact that I published poetry as well as books in political science and psychology drew much negative response. But here, not only is the program multidisciplinary, but so too are the members—it's a unique atmosphere of creativity. A celebration of the program at the end of one academic year featured a flute quartet composed by Ruth Lomon, a composer scholar, and the unveiling of Mary Hamil's new sculpture with ribbons attached containing messages from each one of us. There are also ongoing collaborative projects with members of the Brandeis faculty.

For instance Ruth Lomon has set some of my poems to music, and I planned an event titled "Women Art and Spirituality," featuring Ruth's music, a local poet, and Jane Ring Frank, a scholar who directs and manages the Women's Secessionist Choir in Boston. I have worked a number of times with Susan Dibble, a choreographer and dancer in the Theater Department, on projects around women's issues such as parenting. She created a moving piece depicting her son as a small child accompanying her to her rehearsals.

I also found myself planning events for women's history month every year, working out of my study with the phone and e-mail. It became a satisfying way of weaving my life with that of the program on my own eccentric schedule, discovering I could continue to be present and among the community even if I was not actually on campus.

In fact, if anything, my interests became more compelling. I had a new perspective on human rights since mine were also at stake as a patient and in my attempts to stay socially and professionally connected. As soon as the book on the Mothers appeared, I took up the project I had abandoned when I first traveled to Argentina. I began to interview women of all cultures and backgrounds who had worked on behalf of women's human rights.

This time, I was unable to use the library for my research or to take many trips. My good friend Marilyn Ewer, who has her own business yet manages to find time for volunteering in a number of areas, including Native American rights, offered to do the library work for me. Marilyn happened to be the one friend who stayed close to me in the difficult first years when I was at home feeling adrift and very much alone. She suggested we start our own business with a huge pile of one of my books a press offered to sell me because it was closing. We founded Brewer Press, the name a combination of Ewer and B for Bouvard. She designed flyers and rented mailing lists while I rented a box at the local post office. Because of her, I had a place to go and something to do. My study became the shipping room, and she devoted a corner of a table in her office to press affairs. We actually sold most of the books in a few years and even made a small profit. But the most important thing was her presence in my life, which included her suggestion for a project that lifted me above my perplexing situation.

While Marilyn was spending time at the library for me, I tracked down women whom I wanted to interview as well as conducting research. But now I was able to take only one long trip, and that was across the country to interview Juana Guitierrez, the head of Mothers of East Los Angeles. My friend Heidi lived there as well as my cherished niece Michele, who was teaching at the University of California at the time. I stayed with Heidi, who did everything possible to make me comfortable, and my niece drove me to my interview.

I was amazed by what I found. In the midst of a crime-ridden area were a clean park, buildings unmarked by graffiti, and a vibrant community, thanks to the efforts of the East Los Angeles mothers. When I marveled at what I saw, Juana told me, "The mothers started a telephone chain. As soon as one of us would see a drug dealer on the street we would call each other and then gather outside until there were about forty of us moving towards those people. They ran away and never came back." The mothers then persuaded the police to keep a presence there, not an easy task, and now their children are able to play outdoors in safety. I spent a few hours interviewing Juana and her daughter, who works with her. I was awed at how such a group of women with little education was able to take on the political establishment in California and mobilize hundreds of people to its cause, and excited at how this would inspire students.

But when my niece Michele dropped me off at Heidi's apartment, I was in such a fog of exhaustion that I couldn't sleep. I spent the rest of my day and a half there on her couch or walking in her neighborhood. But I came home with new material, thrilled to have met these women who modeled themselves on the Mothers of the Plaza de Mayo and who had worked successfully to prevent the construction of both a prison and an incinerator that would have burned 125,000 pounds of toxic wastes daily in the mothers' backyards.

Given my fatigue, I knew I could no longer travel for interviews, but I had resources at my disposal. I used my contacts in the human rights community to learn about activists who were traveling to Cambridge and Boston, carefully scanning the travel arrangements of people such as Dai Qing. One of the leading Chinese dissidents, she had criticized the legitimacy of the communist system by her independent historical studies and her journalism, endeavors that were tightly controlled in China. I discovered that she was in New York City en route to be filmed for a documentary. But I also had to deal with the language barrier, for although Dai Qing had a smattering of English it would not be enough for a long interview. I then learned that Zhu Hong, who had spent twenty years in a punitive collective farm doing menial work for her crime of raising questions about the regime while a professor, was actually spending the semester at Boston University. We were the same age, but she walked with her back bowed and with the gait of an elderly woman, a testament to her years of brutal hardship in China. With her help I contacted Dai Qing while she was in New York, paying for her train ticket so that I could interview her at my home. Zhu Hong helped me with the interview, for Dai Qing was more comfortable with Mandarin. After the interview I prepared dinner for Dai, and we spent a wonderful evening laughing and talking as if she had not spent long years trailed by the security police and time in prison.

The Women's Studies Program at Brandeis was yet another way of bringing some of these women to the area. For my book on women and human rights, I wanted to include a range of women, not only those with national reputations but some who had worked locally and against great odds, who were unsung heroines in the broader society. In fact, I decided to dedicate a section of the book, which I titled "Environmental Racism," to women who had worked on the environment, for I now considered a healthy environment a human right. In the process I discovered that the worst toxic wastes were dumped in unsafe conditions in minority and Native American communities. I organized a lecture series at Brandeis on environmental racism, doing something for the Women's Studies Program while facilitating my interviews for a section of the book.

I first contacted Dolly Burwell, an African American woman who was a leader in opposing the dumping of PCBs in rural Warren County, North Carolina, where she lived. In the process of arranging her visit to Brandeis to speak in the lecture series I began researching toxic wastes, landfills, and the racial and socioeconomic nature of communities with hazardous waste sites. It opened me up to a new world and became an interest I would continue to pursue for my own education. Like many women who are activists, Dolly wove her hectic political life with mothering. We spent much time talking about our children and our lives. When she left for the airport to return home, she told me, "I got me a sister."

One of the women I invited to speak and who stayed with me was Grace Thorpe, or No tan oh quai, her native name, which means Big Windy Woman. And that was an apt description, for she was over six feet tall, loud, and very outspoken about her feelings against the storage of nuclear waste in Native American land. The day before her talk, she announced, "I want to go shopping. I need to find a gift for my daughter." I spent an hour and a half sitting on the floor of a department store while she browsed with gusto through an array of cheap jewelry. That afternoon she felt ill from her heart condition, and I spent the afternoon sitting beside her and offering comfort as she lay on our living room couch. She wore me out during her stay, but I will never forget her courage and her many accomplishments. Grace told me how she had given a speech against the storage of nuclear waste from a telephone next to her hospital bed. She became yet another role model for me.

Oddly enough, while I was conducting research on environmental issues and the dangers of toxic wastes, I never suspected that this would later yield an insight into the toxic wastes in our town and the many possible causes of my own illness. Dolly Burwell's words would come to haunt me: "Although areas where poor black folks live have the worst toxic wastes, there is no safety anywhere."

In 1996 my book *Women Reshaping Human Rights: How Extraordinary Activists Are Changing the World* appeared, published by the publisher of my book on the Mothers of the Plaza de Mayo. The book I so wanted to have for my students was finally completed.

As usual my interests shifted, and I began planning an anthology about grandmothers from different cultural backgrounds as well as making significant revisions of the book I had written on grieving. The book *Grandmothers: Granddaughters Remember* was my way of honoring the heroism of my own grandmother, who lived through two world wars, and of illuminating the commonality as well as the unique gifts of people from different ethnic and racial backgrounds. Gestating new projects is like swimming toward buoys in the ocean. It is a way of giving I can no longer do in a classroom situation, as well as a way of exploring the world without traveling.

⌇⌇⌇

Every Tuesday and Thursday scholars in the Women's Studies Program present the results of their research. On the rare occasions when I am able to attend one, there is always a heated discussion along with positive reinforcement, which is the very breath of the program. Even though I need a two-hour nap afterward, I feel renewed and inspired by these sessions.

Recently a scholar who had contracted polio as a child gave a presentation on her work as an activist for the disabled and on her autobiography, drawing a packed audience. She paralleled her coming out and the sense of wholeness she had acquired as a result of her battle with illness and her late awakening to the women's movement, describing both as a revolution. It proved to be an opportunity to speak about my own illness as well as to help people through their perplexity in responding to the disabled.

Afterward, during the discussion—which seemed to skirt the reality of illness—I spoke about the issues of living with invisible disabilities, something I had never done before in such a setting. That may not seem extraordinary to the healthy, but for me it was a political statement about community and mutual understanding, my own gesture of "coming out."

This time I was not addressing hospice workers and ministers but people I saw socially and as colleagues. Hence revealing myself not only as a scholar but also as someone living with a difficult condition was much more demanding and meant cutting through the thickets of my pride as well as ending my silence. It meant that now my illness was no longer a secret except to my close friends. Because I exuded enthusiasm and interest, revealing my physical vulnerability was a personal risk because it tended to make people uneasy. But an unexpected benefit was that, henceforth, I would be able to explain my low attendance at many events and would not only be understood but also respected.

It also gave me an opportunity to help other people. "How do I respond to disabled persons?" a scholar asked after that presentation. "As you do to a human being," I answered with hidden exasperation. Upon reflection, I realized that a very common reaction to ill people is one of puzzlement, as if we were somehow a species apart. The question I found so irritating was really a request for guidance, a plea for how to deal with the awkwardness and discomfort many of us feel when confronted with a distressing situation.

My reply was in effect an acknowledgment that I exist as someone despite my health problems, for all too often conversations leave out that part of myself, making me feel terribly alone. This exchange also served as a spark for my work. In the years to come, it would be the impetus for writing about and giving presentations at Brandeis on various aspects of living with IC.

That afternoon also made me aware that I was learning to ask for consideration of my special needs. When I advise students, for instance, I tell them they must come to my house because of my limitations. For a period, I helped found and edit a new publication of the Women's Studies Program, but I did most of the work at home when I felt well enough. Now my contributions come in the form of electronic mail. More often than not, I have to forgo events I would really like to attend, but I know there is a place for me when I surface, no matter how long I have been absent.

I am grateful to be part of a community, especially one that considers all the scholars as resources. I can do what is close to my heart in ways I would have never dreamed possible. I am once again combining jobs, navigating illness, and pursuing my research and writing. But now I am doing so in the company of women whose range of interests is far more diverse, women I would never have had the opportunity to meet, much less learn from, in my former teaching job.

In fact, my work at the Brandeis Women's Studies Scholars Program has a startling continuity with the peaceful anarchist model of direct democracy the Mothers of the Plaza de Mayo adopted and with my research and writing on women human rights activists. The women activists I studied and interviewed created organizations that functioned in a nonhierarchical and spontaneous way, giving them maximum flexibility. They wove together their public efforts with the skills of their private lives, where managing intimate relationships was so important. Like the Mothers' organization, the Women's Studies Scholars Program operates with a sense of caring and a lack of competition that is quite unusual. How different this setting is from the one I experienced in my former life as a professor.

A friend recently asked me if I missed teaching. I replied that often I dream I am in the classroom but that I would never have had this wonderful opportunity at Brandeis if I were still teaching. "Would you be teaching if you weren't ill?" he asked, and I replied, "Yes, I would be rushing throughout my life without stopping to reflect."

⚹ ⚹ ⚹

One of the problems I encountered in creating a new life for myself was how to translate my reality when talking with friends and acquaintances who enjoyed good health. I discovered that finding space in conversation for the lives of the disabled is part and parcel of working toward human rights. The inability of many people to understand the changes that had occurred in my life was not a matter of ill will but the result of a social discourse that ignores the issues of living with any kind of illness. I had written the first edition of a book on grieving ten years ago because of the confused silence that greeted me after my mother's death. I then discovered that sadness was taboo because it signified loss of control in a society that values it so highly. It took me some years to realize that chronic illness is also a subject that arouses fear and discomfort in many people.

I discovered that I had to negotiate not only my hours very carefully but also my conversations. I would have to learn to speak like a diplomat who deals with people from different countries. I already knew the language of the healthy, but since I came from the country of the disabled, which doesn't wish to be colonized, my only weapon was to forge my own way of speaking. That didn't happen quickly or in an organized way but occurred spontaneously and over time. Often, I thought of what I would have wanted to say after a difficult situation had come and gone.

Because I did not want pity and did not want to risk upsetting anyone, I found myself assuring people that I was managing very well. Similarly, a friend who was recently widowed felt she had to tell others that she and her husband had had a fulfilling and long life together and therefore she was lucky, as if that wonderful bond didn't make the loss of her husband even harder for her.

I am often greeted with the question "How are you?" which is as much a formality as saying hello. I know I am expected to reply, "Fine, thank you," but I am so tired of that ritual of lying that I have learned how to answer with the statement "I am." That seems to be more accurate and requires no explanation.

But unfortunately, as a disabled person I often feel deprived of conversation, not about diagnosis or medical details, not as complaint, but rather of the basic need to tell my story. The hard work of my everyday life is invisible to people who enjoy good health, because they have the very human propensity of taking their ease for granted. It's difficult to share with a healthy person such triumphs as walking around the block or having a pain-free night. I also want to speak about how suffering has transformed me; illness is a school that yields surprising insights.

There are always three stories when I converse with most people and often with family members: their story, my edited story, and my invisible story of climbing the peaks of illness. It is my invisible story that hungers for recognition and acceptance. Often I am caught in a dilemma because, although I don't wish my condition to be the main topic of discussion, I would like to have it acknowledged, however briefly. When it isn't even mentioned, my illness seems to weigh more heavily on me.

I learned that changing the way we speak about the ill, much less giving them room in social discourse, requires drastic and far-reaching efforts to transform cultural attitudes. So much of what we say regarding the disabled stems from deeply held social attitudes. I once listened to a scholar speak of her aunt who had recently lost her vision. "She doesn't do anything. She just stays home and won't even join a group for the blind." As I pondered her reactions, I realized that these conclusions were not just a result of her own observations. Inherent in those comments and in many others I have heard was the socially inspired view that ill people must be heroic and that they must band together, for they are part of a separate group.

Expanding the discourse around illness is not an easy matter, and I found that I needed several approaches to even begin addressing this problem. Since the disability movement is involved in efforts to change public images of the disabled and the vocabulary used when speaking or writing about them, I turned to the more private work of using poetry to speak about illness. It is a quiet effort to create a sense of community that honors and celebrates diversity. Poetry is the ultimate free space where I can speak of what hurts in life and express my passions, moving beyond labels and insisting on my humanity. For instance in a poem entitled "With Giacommetti," I ended with this section: "Poised on chariots, we are tiny / and the wheels are huge. / But we stretch beyond / our height. We devise a taut balance. / Sometimes we sing."

As I was finishing a book project, my friend Marilyn and her partner took me to the De Cordova Museum in Lincoln to see an exhibit of drawings, paintings, and installations by artists who were ill. I was struck by the drawings of an artist who was suffering from AIDS and who represented his body with great eloquence. That exhibit inspired me to complete a cycle of poems I had started at the Virginia Center for the Creative Arts, which became a chapbook titled *The Body's Burning Fields*.[1]

I contacted a close friend of mine, Aileen Callahan, who is an artist, and she and I began a collaboration of drawings and poetry about illness that became an exhibit circulating among medical school galleries in Massachusetts and Ohio where medical personnel pass throughout the day. It was also part of a large symposium and exhibit in Ohio on art and medicine. It was an inroad, a beginning. Poetry and painting can change patterns of thought, creating new social perspectives. I thought of this joint effort as a small step toward healing society and expanding our view of human rights.

When the chapbook of the exhibit's poems and drawings came out, I received a touching letter from a woman who had bought the book: "Your poetry spoke directly to me and gave me hope, knowing I am not alone. So very few understand what long-term pain and suffering does. I read my own experience expressed in your words, even though the actual conditions are different."

In time I began receiving requests from authors wanting to use one of the poems from the chapbook in a book they were writing about living with illness. My poems appeared in books about Alzheimer's and kidney

---

1. M. Bouvard, *The Body's Burning Fields: Poems of Illness and Healing* (Wind Publications, Lexington, Kentucky, 1997).

disease, to name a few, and were anthologized in poetry books about illness.

᠕᠕᠕

In addition to writing poems, I found that using simple phrases when speaking to people who were ill could be very effective. For example, telling someone "I am sorry," in response to a person's pain, is very power-ful. Spoken with feeling, these words signify "I sympathize, I am with you," affirming suffering as well as giving comfort. Many people believe that somehow they need to say something wise, that they must either try to suggest remedies for us or cheer us up. But as in responding to any kind of loss, the simplest phrases, such as, "You don't deserve this" or "It's not fair," are the most comforting.

I have experienced these in the most unexpected places and times as well as from my own family. Once, while making a connection in a busy airport while returning from the Virginia Center for the Creative Arts, I hailed down an electric cart because I couldn't summon the energy to walk from one gate to another. As I stepped into the front seat, an elderly woman put her hand on my shoulder and asked me, "Are you all right?" I choked up with tears at this very welcome sign of recognition and con-cern. "I'm having difficulty, but I'll make it," I answered. When she de-scended at her gate, she once again asked me if I would be all right. "She must have been looking at you very hard," the driver remarked, "because you look just fine to me." What this elderly woman gave me was very precious: an understanding of my situation that made me visible.

Over the years, my family has learned to deal with my new condition in very simple but touching ways. Once when I felt apologetic about my need for naps in the afternoon, my daughter told me, "What's the big deal? Some people go to work, some people nap!" She changed my per-spective with that seemingly offhand comment. Although I understand how much my husband and children want to help improve my situation, I always tell them that just accompanying me with such simple phrases or with a hug is a truly great gift.

At a time when I felt bereft about not being available, because of my need for long naps, my husband responded to me by saying, "You are the sweetest presence." Reminding me of my importance, the way my hus-band does so frequently, brings me back into a society where I often feel I am just "passing." In my previous life I thought of recognition in terms of my work. Now it has become an act of deep meaning, one that encompasses my whole being.

Private conversations with people suffering from terminal illnesses became a new and important path for my social activism, a way of using what I had suffered. In fact, I found myself unconsciously calling people in distress more and more often in order to comfort them and also because I had come to feel so at ease with such situations. The ability to be there for others is one of the unexpected blessings that can be an inextricable part of tragedies.

I would speak to my husband's friend Patrick, who had an advanced case of lung cancer, over the telephone a few times a week. Sometimes he complained about the metallic taste in his mouth from the chemotherapy or the anger he felt about his solitary struggle in the midst of family. I would tell him, "I'm so sorry that you're in such pain, and you are not a burden. When your family takes you to the doctor it makes them feel less powerless." I always asked, "How is today? How bad is the pain?"

Because of my experience with my own condition, I recognized how fatiguing it was for him to speak and made my calls brief, telling him, "Just hang up when you're tired." I acknowledged the hard work of dying, trying to give him the safety to say what he was feeling and reminding him that we are all terminal. We even joked about death. I quipped that I wouldn't have any part of the afterlife if there were no vanilla ice cream there, making him chuckle.

I discovered from my own experience that there is nothing more irritating to someone who is hurting than an attempt to cheer him or her up or to change the subject. An acquaintance with an advanced case of multiple sclerosis telephoned me one morning when she was feeling particularly blue. I surprised her by commenting how often I wished the plane I was traveling on would crash. She answered, "I always wish a bomb would fall on my apartment," and we both laughed at our death fantasies.

It was a relief to speak the truth in a society that fears both the depth of our feelings and physical vulnerability. I remember hearing someone say that "truth is the province of saints and children," meaning that they are exempt from social niceties. But I believe most of us wish to be accepted without our masks.

Although I learned to speak with people in situations similar to or more serious than mine, I still felt that I needed to learn a more systematic way of bridging the conversational gap between the healthy and the ailing. This led me to begin a study of linguistics, a field my daughter Laurence excels in. During one of our visits to her home in London, she introduced me to this new world by taking me to the largest Waterstone's bookstore in London. It had an entire floor of books on all aspects of linguistics, from the scientific to the social. We spent a wonderful morning browsing, and I returned with a pile of new books to weigh down my luggage.

A year of intense study inspired me to prepare and present a seminar at Brandeis on creating a discourse around illness. I didn't expect this topic to draw many people, but when I arrived in the lounge with its long table I found the room jammed, with people sitting against the wall and also standing. The audience included students, therapists, and nonacademics from the town as well as many of the scholars. I was surprised and delighted at the hunger to learn how to address people with disabilities. It was a very reinforcing experience because it encompassed my excitement at entering a new field along with the realization that my experience with illness could be of use to others.

I spoke about the power of reframing sentences. Reframing means rethinking an experience and expanding our perception of it so it can be handled more resourcefully, which in effect means changing a limiting perspective or outlook to one that offers more positive views about ill people's lives and the choices they believe they have. That is very different from controlling a conversation or telling a person what she or he is thinking and feeling. I remember a friend's physician husband telling me, "You are getting better?" at the beginning of a telephone conversation at a time when I was experiencing great pain.

While my presentation was both scholarly and a form of social activism, it helped me to realize just how much my family and friends had helped raise my self-esteem and changed my perspective by their comments. Once, when I complained about the fatigue and pallor in my face, my husband replied, "But you have the most alive expression." That simple phrase shifted my self-image in the most healing ways. Often kind friends would also speak to me in ways that challenged me to change my views of myself. For instance, when I told a good friend that I had had a most difficult week, she responded, "Think of the books you have written on politics and how they have affected people," thus inspiring me to reexamine myself. I have also heard from caring friends, "You accomplish more than most people who are healthy."

Talking about our lives not only reflects our perceptions but can help change them. I share my inner story with my husband, and it is frequently about good moments or hours such as having a period of good work in the morning, or having a truly restful night. He understands that I have a new perspective on time and that I can speak of how I use it in the most celebratory ways.

⁂

One of the joys of my life as a scholar at Brandeis has been the freedom to explore new fields outside political science such as linguistics and to discover the social uses of poetry. Rather than being criticized for not staying in my field, my new projects are welcomed with enthusiasm and much support. They are the fruits of my continual struggles and my efforts to re-create a life. In my scholarly work I am traveling greater distances than I would have as a professor confined to a single field. But while my research was bringing me to ever-changing vistas, my ability to travel was steadily dwindling.

7

A QUESTION OF TRAVEL

A FTER MY books on the Mothers of the Plaza de Mayo and on women and human rights appeared, I had a number of tempting invitations to speak at various universities across the country. The decisions about whether to take such trips became part of an ongoing quarrel between my heart with its unquenchable enthusiasm and my mind and body. I had always pushed myself beyond my limits when I was healthy and felt that there weren't enough hours in the day to attend to all my interests and responsibilities. Now, when faced with pressing physical limits, I still wanted to follow my love of being in new environments where I could relate to different kinds of students. I was not always wise when making these travel plans and spent many days and weeks agonizing over whether I could actually do so while being lured by my wish to still be in a setting I felt was part of my life.

I planned each trip as if I were preparing for a trek to Nepal. In fact, I kept a journal of these times as if I were a mountain climber writing about the perils of fording icy streams rather than sitting in an airport lounge waiting for a commuter flight. Like the climber, I battled exhaustion and was concerned about what lay ahead. I couldn't predict my endurance. I also felt that I was enriching my presentations with all that I learned from living with illness. I was not only offering concepts that helped students map political reality but also speaking about my shifting perspectives about what constitutes a good life. Thus, the rewards of such trips were more than that of awakening young adults. They were affirmations of our common humanity and the possibility of exploring our relationship to the world and to each other in a new way.

In 1995 I was a guest of the Women's Studies Program at the University of Indiana, invited to speak about the Mothers of the Plaza de Mayo.

I forewarned the faculty members about my limitations and scheduled my flight time so that I could rest in the afternoon before giving my talk.

It had been years since I journeyed to this part of the Midwest, and I marveled at the expanse of the landscape, the broad, empty roads, the farms and small towns that unfurled while I chatted with the driver. "How are you Miss?" he asked me. "Where are you coming from?" Having spent part of my childhood in the Midwest, I remembered just how open and friendly people were. After the crowded Northeast, where people rarely spoke to strangers, I felt the thrill of being in a different region—a joy I would never have experienced if I had decided to decline the invitation.

There was an informal faculty dinner before the event. As the professors got up to help themselves from a buffet, I spoke with a number of them. They were chatting among themselves about work and their daily lives and included me in their conversations as if I were one of them and not a special guest—a great relief.

Once in the auditorium where my talk was held, I was happy to be among students again, fielding their questions. They had read my book about the Mothers and asked me, "What are the Mothers doing now that there has been a change in government?"

"They are continuing their struggle to bring the generals responsible for the disappearances to trial, continuing to demonstrate and to write new slogans every year that reveal government duplicity. In fact, they keep branching out into new forms of activism such as opening a café for political discussions and sponsoring a course on human rights at the university in Buenos Aries. Nothing can stop these women, neither fear of the still pervasive security police, nor the fact that many of them are elderly."

But at the reception after my presentation my energy dissipated, and I needed to lean against the wall. I clearly had reached my limit but didn't quite know how I could leave gracefully when so many students were crowding around me eager to talk. None of them knew that I was ill. To my relief, as the crowd thinned one of the professors offered to drive me back to the motel.

When we arrived she turned off the engine and began telling me, "I've just had a double mastectomy. It's so difficult to accept the awful emotional pain and to speak about it. People think that only women with large breasts get cancer, not skinny women like me." I looked at her more closely and saw that she had not had breast implants, a decision I admired. I listened to her with sympathy and understanding as we spent some restorative time speaking about the taboo subject of illness. I could be myself with all my physical vulnerabilities and also give my support to this woman who lived alone and had no one with whom to share her sorrow. She became a friend, and we exchanged letters periodically for the next few years.

The next morning, a student picked me up to drive me to the airport, chatting enthusiastically during the ride. She was moved by the Mothers' story and told me her own as an emigrant from India. But when I arrived, the airport was mobbed and the flight to Boston late. I was distressed by what this would do to my low energy, but nevertheless marveled that I was actually en route like all the other people thronging the waiting room.

The following year I was invited to be the keynote speaker at the Southwest Pacific Women's Studies Conference in Fullerton, California. In my former life I would have written my presentations as easily as the lectures I prepared daily. This time I needed to labor over my talk because by now my fatigue was affecting my memory. Sleep deprivation had a way of making me so forgetful that I needed to write out complete sentences to speak from rather than the sketchy notes I had once used. I was especially worried about my stamina. Accepting such an invitation meant spending the day in an airplane and then a long day afterward beginning with a speech, a panel discussion in the afternoon, a dinner, and a return flight very early the following morning. "You're crazy to do this," my husband told me. But I stubbornly insisted on going ahead with it. I had spent too many months alone in my study. I also yearned for adventure and a change of scene.

A few weeks before my departure, one of the organizers of the conference sent me a beautiful poster and a schedule of events with my presentation prominently featured. I was simultaneously excited and terrified. The night before the trip, I was so nervous I slept very poorly and woke up fatigued. It was raining and foggy. I worried about the airport closing, about making the connection in Dallas. I kept asking myself how I could have insisted on pushing my body beyond its capacity.

My illness had turned me into a worry machine. All through the flight, I imagined the worst scenarios. With only fifty minutes between flights in Dallas, I was convinced I would miss the connection and be forced to take a much later flight that would get me into the Orange County airport in the early morning hours. To most people, the way I fixated on such details seemed excessive. For me, unforeseen complications meant that the physical toll of such journeys would increase.

As we arrived in Dallas thirty minutes late, there was a dense crush of passengers hovering around a single airline representative. When I asked for an electric cart, the representative dismissed me curtly. But a porter standing nearby with a wheelchair overheard the conversation and motioned me to "hop on the chair." He raced me to the gate, and although the plane door was already closed, the woman behind the desk was kind enough to unlock the door and allow me on the plane.

I arrived on time at the John Wayne Airport feeling as if I had journeyed to the ends of the earth. It was late afternoon in Los Angeles. The professor waiting for me chatted amiably as we inched through traffic. She had no idea how weary I was and how delighted that I had actually made it.

The next morning I experienced the first rewarding views of my trek as I walked through the campus to the building where the conference was being held. I smelled gardenias and jacaranda, feasting on the profusion of such beautiful trees and shrubs, on the greens, blues, and purples after the grayness of a Boston April. The students seemed to be everywhere despite the fact that it was a Saturday. It felt wonderful to be in a university environment again.

When I entered the auditorium, I noticed a very mixed audience, professors as well as students, all of them highly diverse ethnically. I was delighted because the topic of my talk was civility and mutual respect among races and ethnic groups. I made a decision at that very moment that I would speak not as the scholar who had been investigating women's legal and philosophic positions on human rights but as an older woman with experience who had some wisdom to offer. This was a drastic change for a woman who always valued sound intellectual analysis above all, and this experience would steer me toward yet another change in my approach to student audiences.

Although I didn't realize it at the time, my use of language was changing rapidly, as were my goals in addressing people. As I stepped up to the podium after the introduction, I studied faces and expressions so that I could get to know this audience and speak to each person, not at them as a collectivity. When I began, the words I had prepared swarmed out of sight, but my voice was clear and carried well. "It's so important to pay attention to mutual respect at a time when our leaders are blaming certain groups such as 'immigrants,' or 'welfare mothers,' names that are freighted with negativity. Power is more complex than most of us believe and we all possess it inherently in our words and in what we chose to do. We can take the initiative and name ourselves—as the African Americans or First Nation peoples or as Hispanic people who call themselves La Raza have done—rather than allowing ourselves to be categorized in labels we do not fit. We can create a language that mirrors our own reality and helps us develop our political and social consciousness."

A dialogue began. "Who among you are immigrants?" I began, raising my own hand. "Do any of you know someone with AIDS?" Too many hands flew up. "Have you noticed how courageous those suffering from AIDS are?" I received a roar of assent. We were breaking down barriers so carefully erected to keep us in our places. Then I took the ultimate risk. "I am chronically ill. I have been writing poetry about my condition. This has both empowered me and helps to educate people about the realities of illness." I stood up in my competence, not as a former professor or as a researcher, but as a person who has struggled and survived. That I did so in such a public forum was a risky yet important step for me, an affirmation that illness is not weakness but another way of living fully. To my surprise, a woman in crutches stood up and said, "Thank you, thank you."

Suddenly it was over. I crossed the campus again for a nap before returning to the afternoon sessions and a panel discussion with the students. Their professor asked me to speak about why I wrote the book, and in so doing I engaged the students in a discussion about values. "We are here to take care of each other and of the world we live in. You should look at yourselves as the future custodians of a just society," a comment I certainly would not have made in class during my past life.

With a typical California spirit of fun, late that afternoon there was a jazz band to celebrate the conference and a raffle to raise money for the Women's Studies Program. I joined in for a few minutes before walking back to the hotel on the edge of the campus. I had journeyed to Nepal and returned exhausted but exhilarated.

That evening a young woman from Radio Pacifica, a station I had never heard of and that I learned was concerned about ecology and radical politics, came to the hotel to interview me. I didn't really want to do this and told her, "I'm tired and I don't have much energy," but she was so eager and interested, promising to keep it short, that I found it hard to say no. Afterward, I had arranged to have dinner with a close friend and radio colleague of my son who was in town. The young woman spotted us, and I introduced her. She pounced on him, talking at top speed about her program while my son's friend calmly listened without saying a word and handed her his card. I giggled to myself at the way so-called radicals were nevertheless attracted to power.

On the return flight, I recorded those two days minute by minute on slips of paper I carried in my purse. I felt like one of my favorite authors, the zoologist George Schaller writing his notes in the Tibetan mountains while sitting in a sleeping bag after an arduous ten-hour day crossing snow-clad slopes. What might seem to be pedestrian events to the healthy represented a triumph for me, proof of my endurance.

After that trip, I knew that these yearly forays were no longer possible for me. Yet the quarrel between desire and possibility raged as strongly as ever. I was not yet ready to let go, and in 1998 I accepted an invitation from the head of the Latin American Studies Program at Gettysburg College to speak about the Mothers of the Plaza de Mayo. I spent weeks negotiating so that my public presentation and the seminar would be scheduled on different days, explaining my dietary problems and my need for rest.

Although my talk was firmed up almost a year in advance, I spent the months prior in a state of great anxiety, wondering whether my body would support this. The stress of worry exacerbated the pain in my bladder and certainly my poor sleep. I asked myself whether the trip was worth all this suffering. This time, I felt as if I was going mountain climbing without climbing shoes, ropes, or maps.

When I was on the flight headed for Gettysburg, I wondered if other passengers knew how lucky they were. They could get on a plane, arrive at their destination, and actually do something afterward. They could come and go without even thinking they were en route, just focusing on their goal.

While riding to Gettysburg from the airport, I was absorbed by the rolling hills, the abandoned barns, and the sense of tragic history emanating from the landscape. Was it my illness that sensitized me to the bloody events that seemed to call out from a supposedly peaceful stretch of fields? I felt the pain of those awful Civil War years as I watched a countryside that seemed as eloquent as the fields of Verdun, France, where so much carnage was translated into eerie silence.

I needed to nap as soon as I arrived at the hotel, requesting a quiet room. "There's no one above you," the receptionist told me. "You'll be just fine." But when I lay down to sleep there were noises of people walking overhead, thumping and banging. I was unable to rest and went right back to the front desk to ask for another room. "There was no one above you," the same receptionist told me. "We keep that room empty because it used to be a hospital during the Civil War." I hadn't imagined those sounds, but by now I had become used to the new perceptions that come from prolonged suffering. In my enforced solitude I had become aware not only of the depths of my immediate surroundings but of a hidden world we pass by in our haste. Thus these experiences seemed normal to me, although I knew nobody would take them seriously if I mentioned them. Certainly my husband didn't when I told him about them later.

The dinner with faculty members and an evening seminar compounded my travel fatigue. A faculty couple from Mississippi met me at the hotel and immediately asked me, "Where are your people from?" I was taken aback until the woman explained, "In the South, it's a custom to find out about a person's family history." This exchange delighted me and reminded me that being in Gettysburg was a bit like being in a different country.

Somehow the seminar passed in a fog. The students asked very few questions, and I realized that they hadn't really done the required reading and were more interested in the spread laid out by their professor. It was actually a relief. I could speak with them personally about my experience with the Mothers, and it was more like an easy conversation than a formal presentation.

The following day, I would have explored this fascinating town had I been healthy. Instead, I remained in my hotel room. I napped, pored over my notes for what seemed like the thirtieth time, and read a P. D. James mystery to conserve my energy. The new room was perfectly quiet.

As usual, when I saw the auditorium crowded with students, I discarded the notes I had worked so hard to prepare and began speaking from the depths of my experience with the Mothers. I poured all my passion and intensity about the significance of the Mothers' work into my talk, and the audience was silent and intent. "Courage and risk taking are intimately entwined and claiming one's conscience is a powerful act. You may wonder what a group of elderly women can accomplish against a military regime but insisting upon human dignity as the Mothers did means to hold on to our beliefs when the political and social environment usurps individual judgment. The Mothers expressed their power in new ways, not by transforming events but by making space to reveal the ethical significance of these events."

"But the generals are not in prison," a student protested, and I replied, "There are many kinds of prison and fear is one of them. The Mothers have just published a book with the aid of *Pagina Doce* [Page Twelve], a popular newspaper, recounting the terrible deeds of the junta leaders. In a country that still does not honor open reporting and that tries to ignore the Mothers' activities, the Mothers continue to publish profiles of the security police and the military in what they refer to as 'The Gallery of Oppressors' on the back page of their monthly newspaper. Thus, they continue to put the generals on trial."

The students' reaction was so enthusiastic that I felt my trip had been worth the physical and emotional toll it took on me. The director of Latin American Studies, who drove me back to the hotel, told me that I was the one person in the lecture series who truly spoke directly to the students' concerns rather than focusing on his or her research. That comment seemed to vindicate an effort that took such a tremendous physical and emotional toll on my health.

But sitting on the small commuter plane back to Boston, I knew that I could no longer take such trips and that I needed to rewrite my life once again. The aftermath of this kind of travel meant too many weeks of fatigue, too many afternoons resting in bed. I had had signs of a need to shift my energy and attention before this, but as in the early years of my illness, it had been easier to ignore my increasing frailty than to face changes. Now I found myself mourning yet another loss, for I had always loved visiting different campuses and reaching out to students. It seemed as if the need for making adjustments in my life was never ending and that once again I had to consider what I would do with my time, my diminishing energy, and where to focus my interests and creativity.

In giving up travel to universities and colleges, I have also relinquished attending academic conferences that are organized around some of my most urgent concerns. Periodically, now, I read of them in the electronic mail that is sent around to all the scholars. I have never really made peace with the fact that I have been cut off from so much that interests me and feel a deep sense of deprivation whenever I read the details of conferences, knowing that even if they are no farther than my own city, I can't attend.

Despite my limitations, I kept dreaming of new projects. I yearned to travel to Croatia and Serbia to research the Women in Black peace movement, whose membership included women of every ethnic group from the former Yugoslav Republic. This group was an important part of an international organization founded by the Mothers of the Plaza de Mayo: the International Gathering of Women and Mothers in Struggle. It would not be a long trip from Trieste, where I visit my family yearly, and one of my cousins who had connections in Croatia offered to help me. I mulled it over month after month, ultimately accepting the fact that there was a huge gap between my enthusiasm and my ability to travel. While I wrestled with my desire to bring their story to an American audience, I remembered that I had inspired my friend and colleague Louise to become active in human rights issues as a scholar and activist on behalf of the Maquiladoras (women working in sweatshops) in Central America. My sorrow was mingled with admiration for her important work, and that helped me to let go.

Although I could no longer attend conferences as a presenter or just as part of the audience, I had developed a way of living with my illness, pushing myself hard to stay as alive as possible, to be among. Perhaps it's a combination of stubbornness, anger, and a burning hope that still drives me. All I know is that living fully as a person with disabilities takes tremendous effort, each moment of every day. That too is a form of travel and a delicate balance.

8

YET ANOTHER TERRITORY

I N 1 9 9 9 I became ill with fibromyalgia, a not unusual phenomenon for women who have IC and live with interrupted sleep. The most prominent symptom of this syndrome is a deep, burning pain felt throughout the body, although it starts in one region such as the neck and shoulders and then spreads over time to other parts of the body. The name *fibromyalgia* means pain in the muscles and in the fibrous connective tissues. Other symptoms include headaches, chronic exhaustion, sleep deprivation, and skin sensitivities. Like my first experiences with IC, these occurred gradually over time so that I brushed them aside as just passing irritants.

The previous spring, I felt an acute pain in my hips when I slept on my side, but I gave no thought to it or to the rashes and headaches that seemed to come and go with such frequency and that I discovered are part of the syndrome.

That same year, while I was in a physician's office discussing another issue, he asked me to "hop on the examining table" because he had a hunch. He applied pressure on several points in my body, and I experienced great pain in the majority of the eighteen areas. "You have the symptoms of fibromyalgia," he concluded. "What does that mean?" I asked him in wonder. "Nothing," he replied. "Those are just symptoms." I had a number of friends who suffered greatly from this illness but, after some days of worry, promptly forgot about that conversation with the doctor.

Oddly enough, the full-blown symptoms appeared after a day when I was able to walk almost as far as I had before the onset of IC. The hike could not have precipitated the illness, because these conditions tend to occur gradually. My husband and I had just returned from our yearly visit to my cousin Maisi and her family in Sistiana, just outside Trieste. At the end of our stay, my cousin persuaded me to visit her homeopathic physician, and I reluctantly agreed just to please her. Dr. Bianci asked me a series of questions that I felt had little to do with my illness, and I responded in a disinterested manner. Afterward he sent me to an herbal apothecary to pick up some medications. I took them halfheartedly, believing they would make no difference.

Once we were back in France, my husband and I went out for our usual truncated hikes. But I felt a renewed energy, and on our first outing I was able to climb almost as high as I could ten years ago. I was ecstatic. Whatever that bitter potion was, it seemed to have worked.

A few days later my hips were aching terribly and my knees burning with a searing pain. The following week, instead of our daily walks my husband and I drove into Lausanne to see an art exhibit. Even standing took an effort; I had to sit down every few minutes.

The museum we visited, the Hermitage, is set in a stunning park on a hill overlooking Lake Geneva. It has alleys of ancient walnut trees and flower gardens cascading down the hill. After our tour of the exhibit and while my husband was taking photos, I rested on a bench beneath those majestic trees. Somehow the panorama of nature, the cedars, walnuts, and the sound of bells floating up from the valley proved a great comfort.

But on the hour-and-a-half drive back to France, I put on my sunglasses and wept quietly, raged quietly. Although my husband was very supportive, I needed to face my sorrow alone, and I spent our last week of vacation in an emotional upheaval.

After we flew back to Boston, I immediately began to learn about this mysterious illness. I had already crossed the border into the country of disabilities and knew I had to be proactive. I got on the Web, downloading several monographs to research fibromyalgia. In one of them, it was referred to as a debilitating musculoskeletal disorder that produces extreme pain and fatigue. Like IC, it involves a cluster of symptoms that are varied, and like IC this illness does not manifest itself in measurable signs such as blood tests. A book by a professor of medicine and director of the University Clinical Research Center at the University of Texas revealed that over ten million people, mostly women, have fibromyalgia (FMS), a far larger number than those who live with the commonly known multiple sclerosis.

The author also pointed out that aluminum toxicity plays a role in this condition because it inhibits the production of energy and blocks the absorption and utilization of phosphates critical to the creation of energy. This would lead me to take a new look at the level of toxic metals in the soil of our town.

Women who suffer from FMS are low in magnesium and serotonin and hence have problems sleeping. I have great difficulty getting through the night, but my husband frequently gives me back rubs that help me drift back to sleep after a period of wakefulness. "I hate to disturb you," I often tell him, and he always answers, "We are in this together." I keep struggling with feeling that I am a burden, yet my husband reassures me that helping me is of primary importance to him. I have come to understand that such gestures as giving me back rubs assuage the feeling of powerlessness that overwhelms him when he sees me struggle with my various symptoms. I also feel extremely fortunate because I have seen how often illness causes tension and anger between couples. In particular, I watched the marriage of my son's best friend fall apart when he developed multiple sclerosis.

The Klonopin I was taking has muscle relaxant properties, and thus I hoped it would help ease the pain in the soft tissues around joints, in my skin, and in organs throughout my body. Not surprisingly fibromyalgia affects the entire nervous system, and the chemical sensitivities I had been experiencing frequently accompany FMS. Like IC, it is a poorly understood syndrome; recent research has pointed to neurological causes. At last, researchers are looking at these illnesses as affecting the entire nervous system instead of as a collection of discrete symptoms.

Ironically, it was only in late 2000, thirteen years after the onset of IC and the year after I became ill with fibromyalgia, that I read an article in the journal of the Interstitial Cystitis Association, "Seeing the Forest through the Trees," discussing the interrelationships between sensitive skin, FMS, and many other related conditions. The article concluded by stating that few IC and FMS patients find physicians who are aware of the big picture and acknowledged the frustrations patients have experienced when consulting specialists, who tend to focus on their particular area of interest. I thought of the fine book by the cardiologist Dr. Bernard Lown, *The Lost Art of Healing*, stressing the amount a physician can learn from a patient just by listening. Ruefully, I remembered all the times my observations had been brushed aside during a consultation.

Like so many people who are chronically ill or who face what seems to be insuperable difficulties, I continually struggled with the cause of my puzzling array of conditions. This led me not only to begin reading about my illness but also to expand the research I had done for my book on women and human rights, in particular the effect of the environment on health. There are now many elements under discussion as possible sources of interstitial cystitis, such as "toxic insult" (exposure to harmful chemicals in the environment) and viruses. Some researchers are exploring the molecular mechanisms of autoimmune diseases with a view to discovering why 80 percent of those who are susceptible to immune disorders are women.

The specialist I see for interstitial cystitis is especially concerned about the possibility of "toxic insult" and tells me not to drink tap water or eat food with chemical additives. He often comments on the rising number of cancer cases he sees in his practice and on his brother's severe reaction to the chemicals he works with in the construction industry.

My physician's warnings and my conversations with Dr. Schiff suggested that environment and diet might account for the growing number of cancer cases. In her book *Living Downstream*, the ecologist-biologist Sandra Steingraber writes about her and her adopted family's bouts with cancer and the toxicity she believes caused it. She stresses that she was adopted, because genetics is now considered to be only one factor in determining who develops cancer.

During the early period of my illness I was having dinner with colleagues, among them a woman who had spent a year teaching in the Czech Republic. "There were so many people with bladder diseases, I couldn't get over it," she commented, and in the same breath spoke about the environmental hazards she had witnessed. I barely paid attention to this remark, but it would surface years later when I came into contact with so many people who had IC.

When I was conducting the research for my book on women and human rights, which included the right to a healthy environment, I focused on the problem of storing and dumping agents that are considered carcinogenic, such as dioxin and PCBs, in communities where ethnic minorities lived. Somehow I still didn't make the connection between my own condition and what was happening to the population in the areas I was studying.

But on March 26, 2001, Bill Moyers's two-hour documentary on how major petrochemical industries have been concealing the toxicity of their products and their effect on consumers was a groundbreaking sequel to Sandra Steingraber's clarion call in her book. Moyers interviewed lawyers who had amassed roomfuls of company documents, as well as historians of those documents, prominent physicians, and a former official of the Occupational Safety and Health and Administration (OSHA). Among the many dispiriting but not very surprising revelations were examples of how these industries used their economic power to influence the U.S. Congress and the executive branch not only through lobbying but also through political action groups and very expensive and effective public relations campaigns. Of all the thousands of chemicals released into the air and water yearly, including those we use in our homes, only 43 percent have been tested for their effects on health. There are no data at all on the long-term effects of most chemicals on our population.

Watching that program brought back my first view of the strange, blue-green, almost phosphorescent patches around Lake Waban when we moved to Wellesley and my puzzlement over what they were. It was only twenty years later that the environmental organization Greenpeace put up signs warning passersby of lead and cadmium deposits. Only recently did the Massachusetts Department of Environmental Protection enclose the area and post warning signs because of the presence of lead, cadmium, and arsenic. But a simple chain-link fence will not prevent contaminants in the soil from moving inexorably toward the water.

I observed another pond in the town forest curdle and die from deposits of paint thinner a factory had dumped there many years ago. The toxic spill that supposedly caused so many deaths from leukemia in Woburn has slowly and inexorably moved into Wellesley, nearing our wells, for soil travels. There are a number of other spills moving through the town's soil, including a TCE plume that has been found at concentrations double the upper limit of micrograms per liter established by the Environmental Protection Agency. TCE (trichloroethylene) is a solvent known to cause cancer in humans.

Not surprisingly, cancer has taken its toll in our town and our neighborhood. Within a radius of two or three blocks, I witnessed a teenager die of brain cancer, two women of breast cancer, a man of liver cancer, and another man of leukemia. Two families who lived in the same house each had a death from cancer, and one of those families also had a teenager who had uterine cancer and will never be able to have children. I suspect that somehow my illness is connected to this situation. The possibility of such a link was corroborated by a study conducted by the Mt. Sinai teaching hospital in New York City in 2003 and by the Environmental

Working Group.[1] It listed toxic metals in the environment causing a variety of ailments including neurological disorders. Cadmium was identified as the most toxic of metals.

When a bone density test revealed that I had a severe case of osteoporosis in my spine and hip, and I then developed asthma, I was even more convinced that my various conditions were partly environmentally related, for I had always walked regularly, taken estrogen and calcium, and had no family history of either disease. As he handed me the test results, Dr. Bordiuk suggested I read a book on osteoporosis by Alan R. Gaby, M.D.[2] I immediately went out to buy it and found that, according to the author, lead, cadmium, and aluminum cause bone loss. Interestingly, Dr. Gaby also corroborated the findings in the book I had read about fibromyalgia, revealing that magnesium is successful in treating FMS because it plays a key role in blocking the effects of aluminum in the body. Aluminum seems to be ubiquitous not only in the environment but also in antiperspirants and cookware.

When my husband and I are in France visiting family, we usually gather in Switzerland. It's where I have my bladder instillations of Cystistat, at a urology clinic run by the son of a childhood friend. The urologist has told me he knows of no cases of IC in his country, although it is widespread in Europe. I found that fact yet another support for believing that the environment is one of the many causes of this perplexing condition.

Scientists are just beginning to study the relation between the environment and chronic illnesses. These diseases are not apt to capture public attention or funding, because they are still baffling to members of the medical profession and because there are no commonly known cures. But the growing number of people who suffer from chronic conditions points to the environment as one of many important sources. An image from a nature program about pollution I once saw on public television has haunted me for years: an eagle perched on a telephone pole, his wings flapping helplessly, his intricate nervous system shattered.

Keeping myself informed helps me to feel less powerless and gives me an outlet for my seemingly unquenchable enthusiasm for political activism. Once a year I give a lecture on the environment to professor Laura

---

1. Environmental Working Group, *Body Burden* (1436 U. Street N.W., Washington, D.C., 2003).
2. A. R. Gaby, M.D, *Preventing and Reversing Osteoporosis* (Prima Publishing, Roseville, California, 1994), 204.

Golden's class at Brandeis. I speak about the connections between illness and toxicity as well as the importance of nature in our lives and how it has influenced my poetry. I am also part of a pesticide awareness movement in our town. Even though these are small gestures, I have come to see them as having a ripple effect in the public consciousness.

꒰ ꒰ ꒰

I did see an alternative physician for help with FMS, and he prescribed the hormone DHEA (dehydroepiandrosterone), which is supposed to give me energy. "There's not much else I can do for you," he said. It would take three more years before I saw a physician who would educate me about daily stretching exercises and ice packs to help reduce some of the symptoms of this disease.

The extreme discomfort in my hips, shoulders, and neck made me feel as if my body were engaged in endless guerrilla warfare—surprise attacks and sudden pauses. The fatigue that accompanies this syndrome further restricted my activities. I was profoundly discouraged. Even though I knew how to handle pain and had years of meditation behind me, I felt that I could never have imagined these new trials. It hurt to take a short walk or even to stand for more than a few minutes. Ironically, I thought I was unlucky to have IC and an autoimmune disorder, but in fact I was blessed to be able to walk with only the limits of fatigue. I thought I had hit bottom but discovered that there is always another layer below.

In order to cope with this new condition I continued my walks, now much shorter and slower. Thirty minutes has been a big triumph and fifteen more the norm. Although he is very athletic, my husband does not mind walking at my pace and waiting during my frequent rest stops. In fact, he always reminds me not to push myself and to listen to my body. But this new restriction makes me feel that I am holding him back, especially when we are traveling.

Walking had always been an important part of my life. While at writers' retreats, my rambles became an extension of my work as I continued to mull over my projects and absorb the landscape. At home I used to walk the two miles into town to run errands, and I walked in the neighborhood to stretch my legs after a long period of sitting at my desk. It was something I took for granted. The streets winding through our section of town were like an extension of our yard; I came to know every tree, house, and even the dogs, which would either bark or welcome me with a wagging tail. Recently, while running an errand, I met one of my neighbors, and she asked me, "I haven't seen you walking in such a long time—where have you been?" "I have fibromyalgia," I answered her, and she was tactful enough to express dismay instead of retreating into embarrassed silence.

Hiking with my husband was always important to our vacations in our mountain retreat. We would climb for an hour or two to reach the most exquisite views over the valley, watching the distant peaks unfold like waves. Now we drive as far up the mountain as possible and amble along cow paths, where there is still a vista if not the spectacle of our higher treks.

Bicycling and ice dancing were also a part of my life. I was not very good at either sport, but I loved the feeling of pedaling up the hills bordering our town or the sensation of flying when I skimmed over the ice, speeding up to make a turn. I'm not a city person and have always felt a need for physical space where I could lose myself. Now it seemed as if I was living in a continually shrinking environment. Sometimes I still dreamed that I was gliding over the ice.

How I appeared to others became a new issue for me. Once, while strolling in a wooded area with some cousins we met in France, I needed to stop and rest on a fallen log. "It looks like a rocking chair," my cousin joked. I was furious and responded, "No, I don't do rocking chairs. Think of it as a motorcycle." As a result of the pain and fatigue of this illness, I have become hypersensitive and catch myself bristling at the most well-intentioned comments.

Errands became another hurdle for me. When there is a line at the cash register in a store, I usually ask for a chair or anyplace where I can sit down, but it's often difficult to find. Once, while shopping for my little granddaughter, I squeezed myself into a kiddie chair that was on display, feeling grateful to be skinny. Sometimes while preparing dinner I sit on a stool by the sink to clean or chop vegetables.

Then there is the issue of traveling: I used to take electric carts to move between gates in airports, but with the advent of long security lines after September 11, 2001, I have had to resort to wheelchairs. Being pushed in a chair emphasized the difference between myself and the people who rushed by as if walking were a given and not a privilege.

Entertaining friends for dinner had always been a great pleasure for me. I would prepare a meal slowly and in increments throughout the day to conserve my energy and to be able to enjoy the evening. I now limit these invitations to close family and only rarely to our friends.

One of the characteristics of FMS is its utter unpredictability. Perhaps twice a year I have a day or two when I am able to walk without pain and at a brisk (for me) pace. Then I think to myself, Oh the things we take for granted in this life until they are taken from us: sleep, feeling well, lack of pain, mobility.

꙳ ꙳ ꙳

I knew I would have to change my lifestyle and thought of the word *revise*, a very powerful word for a writer. It means improving a work in progress. It meant, in my situation, that I would have a choice and that I would continue to live well but in different ways. When people tell me that I've done so much in the past I should rest on what I've done, I say to myself, "I live in the present. Although it is what has made me, the past is not enough."

I scaled down some of my efforts, finding them nonetheless rewarding. The year after I came down with FMS, a researcher for a documentary film company contacted me regarding a film on the Million Mom March for Gun Control that took place in 2000. She had read my book about the Mothers of the Plaza de Mayo and wanted to include some photographs in the film. It was the beginning of yet another project, as I sent out some unedited videos I had brought back from Argentina that would become part of that film along with my comments on the first takes of the documentary on the Million Mom March. I may have spent one hour on the telephone with this woman and even less time on e-mail or looking at her videotape, but I learned that an hour or two can be richer than days spent on routine matters.

There are also an infinite number of possibilities within the Brandeis Women's Studies community. I am in the midst of collaborating with an artist and sculptress with whom I have previously worked. Karen Klein has sculpted parts of discarded trees into fantastic and resonant pieces. I wrote poems to accompany each one for a show called The Intimate Lives of Trees. Because of my energy level, she mailed me photos of her pieces, but I also spent two wonderful mornings sitting in her studio inhaling the smell of resin and letting the sweep of her bold sculptures take hold of my imagination. This is a project that moves me deeply because I see it as an opportunity to influence societal views of beauty, especially to celebrate the wounded and aging body. We exhibited in the gallery at the Women's Studies Research Center and later in the Natick Library. Our collaboration—a celebration of the allure and depth in fragility—drew an enthusiastic response.

I also wanted to explore, with the leader of the research group on women's health that I am part of, my changing views of what constitutes work. I designed an afternoon event with a panel of scholars discussing the surprisingly expanded definition of "occupations." One of the panelists described her recovery from breast cancer as a special kind of work. As a result of the initial constrictions of my life, I have come to realize how much of life's opportunities lie in our immediate surroundings. I don't need to go to distant holy places to find God or to travel to share my projects. My illness keeps requiring that I rearrange my life. While there are long periods of frustration and grief when I do so, such times are also gestations.

Folded into that lesson is a new respect for the way so much of my work is accomplished, seemingly in fragments and at odd moments. One night during a waking moment, for instance, I revised a poem that had been bothering me for some time. There is something reassuring in those moments, for, like my nights, writing is a perilous journey, and yet these insights come when I am the most ill at ease. Is there a connection between the ability to create and giving oneself up to landscapes without maps, to experiences without frameworks, to periods without meaning?

Once, while my husband was standing on line at the grocery store and I was waiting in the car, I found myself scribbling notes for a new project on half of an envelope I had in my purse. Ideas will pour forth while I am taking a walk and am seemingly absorbed in the trees, the shrubbery in front of houses, either enjoying the warmth of the sun or braving a chill wind. I have found that my work is like an underground river that surfaces at odd times and places but is always in motion. Continuing to keep a journal to mark the triumphs and my anguish is also a way of moving forward when it seems as if I am standing still, a way of reaching toward meaning as well as self-discovery. It is something I can do under the worst of circumstances.

᠀ ᠀ ᠀

The onset of fibromyalgia seemed to make my writing much more important to me and helped me discover that there is no distinction between my writing and my life. Slowing down has meant noticing my surroundings with a new depth and awareness. It was as if I were walking a mountain path, examining each wildflower or exposed root and fallen trees instead of speeding to the top.

Shortly before the onset of IC, I decided that I would write only about what fired my soul; even though I was dedicated to research, the process and work would aim to reach an audience beyond academia. That decision made me toss out a scholarly manuscript on grief. While my research remained the foundation for the book, I rewrote it as if I were addressing each reader personally. By hindsight, I was already on the road to changing my life.

Writing has become a layering of experiences: excitement and delight on the one hand, and now, with this new illness, battling the tedium of exhaustion and a mind slowed by medication and pain on the other. I slog through pages over and over again, often wrestling with an intellect that seems to have lost its keenness and facility. However, completing the books helps eliminate the thought "It's not possible." Most important, even though I have so little time to write, the books and poems are in the forefront of my thoughts at odd times throughout the day and even during my waking moments at night. I no longer have to put them aside continually for my teaching.

Every few years I am still able to travel to the Virginia Center for the Creative Arts for the opportunity to focus on my writing without interruption. This is one area of my life where I have experienced a sense of continuity, since I have had many residencies there. I feel lucky because it happens to be the one retreat in this country that accommodates people with health problems. It is also the place where I write most of my poetry, and since the onset of my illnesses I have published two books and two chapbooks of poems.

During my last residency there was a woman writer suffering from post-polio syndrome. The staff made every effort to accommodate her needs. But most of all she and I were part of the group of visiting artists and not made to feel "different." When there was a party with dancing one evening, one of the painters took her wheelchair and pushed it around the room in time to the music. Another evening, the artists held a late-night party in the studios rather than in the residence because they knew I needed to retire early.

I am always given a quiet studio where I can rest afternoons and, whenever possible, one of the two rooms with a private bath, which are usually reserved for couples or visiting members of the board of directors. Although artists are not permitted to request special meals, because of budgetary concerns, the center's cook always manages to find something I can eat, and I take the center's van to the supermarket so I can buy provisions for lunch. One of the administrators of the center, Sheila

Gulley Pleasants, arranges this for me as if it were a routine matter, never making me feel as if I were a burden. When I thanked her for this consideration, she once replied, "We need Marguerite here."

While I invariably experience weeks of travel anxiety beforehand, and the ensuing fatigue, I am always delighted to be in a landscape that I have come to love, with its profusion of trees, its open fields, and quiet back roads. I usually go there in April, when the weather swings from one extreme to another, but invariably the weeping cherries spread their luscious veils and I work in a silence that is punctuated only by birds. Once I am settled in my studio in the beautifully articulated barn that houses us all, I feel the creative energy that surrounds me. There is a rule that no one should interrupt any of the artists while they are in their studios, yet our solitude takes place in an atmosphere of mutual support and sharing. There are open studios and readings on many evenings, events I would never be able to attend at home. Sometimes during the lunch hour I visit the artists' studios to see their work in progress, listen to the composers' tapes, and feel I am nourishing my soul.

The years I am unable to travel to Virginia, I sometimes drive to Provincetown during the winter months, when the rents are cheap, for it is only an hour and a half away from my home. I do so to concentrate on my writing but also to express my autonomy. I have always been independent and fear becoming overly reliant on those I love. I rent the lower half of an artist's home that has a row of windows and a small jetty over the water. Here my days become seamless as I write, daydream, or drive to a nearby cove to gaze at the gulls careening over the sand, immersing myself in my projects and in the measureless spaces of the ocean. My neighbor works upstairs, and her creativity and concentration are part of the swishing tides that seem to enter the room where I sit hunched over my laptop, the dark interior smelling of old wood, and I revel in the meditative routine of living in my writing project. Her dining room is above the kitchen, and I can hear the telephone and wafts of conversation, feeling that I am in company while enjoying my privacy.

Once while I was there I revised the book I had written on coping with grief to include new chapters, especially about mourning a death from AIDS. While previously I had traveled for my research, now, for this revision—with the enthusiastic help of my physician daughter-in-law Mary and my niece Michele—I interviewed people around the country by telephone. I had so many interviews lined up that I spent many hours talking with bereaved fathers, mothers, sisters, and lovers. I was also mourning the loss of a young friend who was a ballet dancer in the Paris Opera Corps de Ballet, and he moved through the pages. When I finally finished that part of the book, I noted in my journal: *This section is a miracle. People shared their sorrow with me, gave me their stories unstintingly as gifts. Our grief is made of so many different strands, has carved a well where others can drink. It was very moving to discover how such a terrible loss transformed the survivors, as if their world had suddenly opened and gained new significance. Transformed by our pain, perfect strangers spoke to each other's hearts as if we were one great heart beating in concert.*

Somehow, in the chaos and unpredictability of my life, the books get written, and one follows another. Liberated from the strictures of being associated with one academic department, I explore fields I would never have considered before, such as linguistics. My career as a writer does not represent a continuum. Rather it is like the growth of an apple tree I once admired in the Virginia landscape. Its trunk seemed to veer in all directions as if it had begun on its knees steeped in meditation, then rocked backward, its limbs reaching outward in a spiral that seemed to turn back toward its base. I saw in this tree the endless braiding of the self that escapes easy definition. Since it was still in the early days of spring before the tree had begun to foliate, I also saw that it was the process, and not the flowers or leaves, that mattered and that this risk taking was what had helped me develop endurance. Writing will continue to be the center of my life regardless of my struggle with fibromyalgia, and new interests will always inspire me to begin yet another book or article.

9

HONORING THE BODY

FINDING proper medical care for my various symptoms is ongoing work. In 2001 the urology practice where I received my monthly instillations fell apart, and the physician's assistant, Lisa Cautillo, was laid off. It was a great blow because of the special treatment she had always given me. I mourned her departure, and while I searched for another practice I telephoned her frequently, for she felt as bad as I did.

Then a friend suggested I consult a urologist who lived closer to our home and practiced at the Newton-Wellesley Hospital. It was an unfortunate choice. When I came for my appointment, there were so many people waiting for him that there weren't enough chairs. As the time passed, I noticed that his patients came in and out as if through a revolving door. When my turn came, I was unprepared for what was coming. He said, "Undress," without looking at me. Instead of following the usual procedures of applying Betadine to prevent infection and a numbing gel, he pushed the catheter into my urethra with such unnecessary force that I cried out. He didn't stop or respond but kept pushing. That was my five-minute visit.

I came home in blinding pain, and when it didn't subside after a few days I called his office. He didn't return my calls at first, and then my husband contacted him. The physician's only response was to suggest I had a bladder infection. I became so uneasy I consulted one of my former urologists, who performed a cystoscopy on me, discovering that the way the catheter was jammed into me had caused a fissure in my urethra. For the next six months I needed to sit on an inflatable rubber tube.

The pain was difficult to bear, but my feeling of anger was worse. I had been treated like an object, like an anonymous organ on a long assembly line of parts unattached to human beings. I wrote an outraged letter of complaint to the physician in question, knowing I wouldn't get a response and feeling overwhelmed with a new sense of powerlessness.

I then called the Interstitial Cystitis Association for a list of urologists practicing in my area. I felt less alone when the young woman I spoke to assured me that she received many phone calls from women experiencing difficulties with physicians.

This experience was yet another lesson. Before deciding on a new urologist, I interviewed his secretary over the telephone to find out whether a commonly used numbing gel, Lidocaine, was used for bladder instillations as well as an antigravity tube that provides a slower and more comfortable procedure. My experience at the Newton-Wellesley Hospital had taught me that these were not givens. Luckily, after a number of unsuccessful visits, I found a physician willing to work with me who took time from his busy schedule to inquire how I was feeling. Dr. Church was not only courteous but also managed to ignore the anger I exuded over the trauma to my urethra during our first few visits. I was tense and defensive, but his easy manner helped me relax.

The following year, my daughter-in-law, Mary, decided to step in and help me organize my care. She telephoned Dr. Kristene Whitmore, a urologist with a national reputation who founded a practice at the Graduate Hospital in Philadelphia that was unique for its holistic approach. Because of her physician status, Mary was able to get me an appointment within a month of her call. My husband and I made hotel arrangements, and we drove down from Boston on a blustery winter day. After my previous experiences I didn't have much hope, but the visit proved to be a revelation.

While I sat in my johnny waiting for Dr. Whitmore, an energetic blonde woman in a leopard-skin top and cowboy boots came bustling in and greeted me with a radiant smile. She covered every one of my physical problems and made recommendations, suggesting topical use of Estrace cream to help heal my urethra. Immediately afterward I saw a physician who dealt with vulvar pain and a young woman who was an expert in dealing with stress. The following morning I went to a physical therapist who works with Dr. Whitmore and who evaluated my musculoskeletal structure and taught me exercises to help ease the pain of fibromyalgia. That afternoon I met with a man who heads yet another type of physical therapy for patients with urological problems and who gave me sacro-cranial massage. I had never heard of such therapy, which focused on my sacroiliac and also on parts of my head. It proved so helpful that I scheduled a return appointment.

This was the first time in my long years of illness that I could discuss all my problems in one setting where they were viewed as interrelated. In fact, when Dr. Whitmore was reading my chart and noticed that I had asthma, she said, "Is that under control or do you need help with it?"

When we returned I began a program of myofascial massage for fibromyalgia pain that Dr. Whitmore had suggested. I happily created a new folder in my file cabinet. Right next to the one labeled medical I wrote "Whole Body Care."

I liked the term *whole body*. Finally, a physician had considered me in my entirety, and that helped my battered self-image. An important part of my self-care then became to honor the body I so often regarded as a betrayer. Since the onset of fibromyalgia, the walks with my husband I loved so much had become slower and very painful. As the joggers passed us during our trek around Lake Waban, I saw them as winged beings and myself as a snail.

This made me realize just how much my self-image was subtly influenced by comparing myself with others and by the way society views the disabled. The times I was in a wheelchair at an airport, I often saw people staring at me, and I felt a deep humiliation. Although the disabilities movement has made great strides toward including the disabled in the broader society, I found that most people are still very uncomfortable at the sight of wheelchairs, leg braces, or a person with a guide dog.

As a woman with disabilities, I have become very sensitive to social images and responses to people like myself. For example, I always admired the political comedian Russell Baker until I heard him parody the idea of putting up a statue for Franklin Delano Roosevelt sitting in his wheelchair. "You have to be PC [politically correct] these days," he grinned. I was shocked by his insensitivity and by the way the audience burst into laughter at his supposed humor.

His comments reminded me of the time my friend Eva, a human rights lawyer who happens to be blind, was interviewed on the television program 20/20. She told me that as soon as the cameraman and the anchor saw her guide dog, the camera was rarely turned on her. People might wonder how she knew, but Eva had developed very keen perceptions as a result of losing her sight. The irony in both stories is that what was at stake was not Eva's blindness or President Roosevelt's partial paralysis but our own inability to consider her as a lawyer or to see Roosevelt's wheelchair as a means of transportation, not as a source of shame.

Because of these experiences I was deeply moved when the artist and model Matshuka posed for the front cover of the *New York Times Magazine* with the scar from her recent mastectomy prominently displayed. It was a socially provocative act but one I thought was long overdue. I saw myself in that photo and felt empowered. Yet I sensed that if the photographer hadn't deliberately made the lighting soft and arranged her dress in a graceful flow, her portrait would never have appeared on the front page. I found that the revelation of a terrible scar on a beautiful woman opened a window on the depth and contradiction of the human experience.

I remembered my neighbor Ernie and also a very dear male friend who both became bald as a result of chemotherapy and decided to forgo wigs. They didn't wish to be disguised and were making an important, unspoken statement that reflected my deeply held wish: "We are still whole, still part of."

One afternoon, when I was driving into Boston for my monthly bladder instillation, I had an unexplained vision that altered my perspective in the most astonishing way. From my car window I saw a man struggling with a walker along an empty sidewalk. For a brief moment that sidewalk became a stage, and the man's struggle assumed epic proportions. It was as if I were seeing the awful dignity and divinity of the human condition writ large. The people hurrying farther down the street suddenly seemed much smaller.

He represented what I had learned about the body in distress, that suffering can be the source of profound learning, helping us to develop compassion and understanding and to realize our humanity. According to Buddhist thought, the unawakened try to deny suffering in life and to pretend it has nothing to do with them. Such denial is futile because no one is really immune to pain. If we close our hearts and minds to the distress around us, we are locked into an undeveloped version of ourselves, incapable of growth and spiritual awakening.

My condition has given me a new understanding of what is beautiful. I keep a photo on my desk of a Russian icon of Saint John in the desert, a skinny, angular figure that seems to bear all the wounds of the world as well as a deep knowing. I also think of the discarded trees that Karen shaped into such strong presences for our project The Intimate Lives of

Trees, and how they celebrate the richness of lives in distress, at the same time breaking down the taboos against age and frailty.

One of my friends who has had breast cancer wrote to me recently telling me that her illness heightened her sense of community: "In an age known for 'cocooning' I have experienced a deep sense of community among those sharing serious illness, one not of shared misery, but of shared courage."

✴ ✴ ✴

The time I devote to minding my body is not only for alleviating my symptoms but also for enabling me to pursue my passions and maintain the quality of my life. Mornings, I spend fifteen minutes doing stretch exercises that I learned in Philadelphia and lifting two-pound weights, my version of "pumping iron." Whenever possible, I take short walks and try to meditate evenings before preparing dinner. Treating my body/mind with respect and attention is an important part of my work of illness. So is the endless amount of time I spend coordinating my care between various physicians, doing research on chronic illnesses, and keeping abreast of new developments in the treatment of IC and fibromyalgia.

I am now undertaking what is often a very difficult lesson for people in this culture: learning to listen to my body's needs rather than making lists of action items, accepting rather than continually attempting to control. When I enter a particularly trying phase that may come without warning or for no apparent reason, I have to put aside my plans and redirect my efforts. These periods of enforced rest have helped me to develop yet another perspective on time and productivity: I am learning how to surrender to my body's cues rather than ignoring them.

Rest is thus an important part of this task. For me, it used to signify an absence. Over the years my therapist had frequently reminded me "resting is hard work." Now I consider it as an activity, a focusing on regenerating my body. Because I am always fizzing with ideas and projects, rest is an extremely difficult undertaking for me. I try to think of myself as in training during these periods, like a mountain climber preparing for a difficult trek.

Another aspect of honoring my body is learning how to ask for help without feeling that I am a burden, although I keep telling people that receiving is as much a way of grace as is giving. It has been very difficult for me to cut through the thickets of pride, independence, and denial, because I am used to being the one who is giving. But I am very fortunate, for now that my husband works at home he has started doing the grocery shopping and running errands for me so I can conserve my energy for my writing. One of the hardest things for me is to see myself as a burden. When I tell him this, he reminds me that I used to carry most of the work of child rearing when our children were young and that now it is his turn to pitch in. He often lets me know that I am not imposing on him, and I feel very lucky. When I look at our life together as a whole, I realize that we have created a new division of labor, a new collaboration in our married and in our family life.

Just as I have to navigate the day physically, deciding how to spend my time, I have to continually revise my relations with friends, often calling off appointments and events. My stomach always lurches when I must do so, and I often feel like a betrayer, but my husband reminds me that this is my time now, that I have had long years of giving and that my health and creativity come first. This may sound like a simple thing, but it is the subject of much anguish and self-questioning. I have that very human resistance to change, especially when it may seem like a step backward even though it is actually progress. I still have too many times when my enthusiasm outstrips my resources. I will attend an event at Brandeis that lasts longer than I can manage, meet with a colleague for more than two hours, or support a friend who has problems only to find myself out of commission for the next few days.

Frequently, I have to tell friends, "I can't." There are those who understand, and I am very grateful to have them in my life. I am fortunate to have friends like Heidi, who is a veteran hiker but who always stops periodically when we are walking together without my ever having to tell her that I need to rest, or my former colleague Ana, who makes her telephone conversations short because she knows I tire easily.

I have found that such sensitivity is the exception, for I have a number of friends who are so uncomfortable with my situation that they can neither talk about it nor acknowledge it when we make plans. Added to their unease is the fact that it is difficult to understand my limitations because I look no different from the healthy, aside from my extreme thinness. Once, when I told a neighbor I couldn't visit her because I wasn't feeling well, she looked at me in an ironic way and said, "I think you are just looking for attention, because you look fine." I shot back, "That was a low blow," and she remained silent. In a few cases I have had to break off some long-standing relationships with a heavy heart; on the other hand I am grateful for those I have, and for the acceptance I am given.

But too often, when I traverse difficult periods, I feel my isolation all too keenly.

I remember having arranged to meet an acquaintance from California, whom I hadn't seen for years. I knew I wouldn't have this opportunity again, but as my husband and I drove home from a morning visit to his friends, I realized I had already spent my day's energy and I called off the meeting. Fortunately, she was responsive to my dilemma. Her understanding, along with my feeling of having taken charge of my situation, helped me toward a refreshing, if long, nap and a very restful evening. Most of all, while it seemed as if I had been denying myself something, I was learning how to give back to my body. Every day I face the challenge of finding a balance between what I would like to do and what my body will support.

❧❧❧

Quilting became yet another way of honoring my body. It is a pastime I once shared with my artist mother, who drew the templates freehand for me when she came for weekend visits. All I had to do was tell her the vision in my head, and the design emerged from her hands. It was a way for us to converse without words. When she died, I couldn't pick up the quilt I was working on for a year. I felt as if our closeness and conversation had been interrupted. I know now that we can never be separated and that I am communicating with her in a very deep way when I gather my hoop, needles, and thread.

Sewing was an important part of my childhood world. I grew up listening to the roar of my mother's sewing machine as her skilled hands guided the fabric through the presser foot with top speed and wonders spilled out of that tiny portable Singer.

Before I became ill, planning a quilt was a way of dealing with a difficult working situation. Although I loved teaching, I had great difficulty with the chair of my department, who not only disliked women but would continually try to undermine my courses. I also had uneasy relations with the president of the college. What carried me through was going to a local fabric store and walking through the aisles, looking at colors and buying pieces that would be part of future creations. I would lay them down on the floor of my study while I was preparing lectures. It was a way of rising above a situation I couldn't change. It was also an unconscious realization that small pleasures are healing.

Quilting is a country I can visit for the sheer tactile delight of drawing the thread through the fabric, for I now prefer to work by hand, using the sewing machine only for borders and the backing. I like the suppleness of hand-sewn quilts, but working by hand is also a personal statement. I will take years to make something beautiful in a society that pressures us to run through our days at top speed. It is a way of savoring the present. At any time of day or night I can settle into the wonderful country where time doesn't matter, only color, touch, and beauty.

Now, when I go through one of my dark tunnels, I leaf through my quilting books, plan new designs during the times I am awake at night, think about them when I am in pain. Unconsciously, since my illness, I have always included birds in flight, either on the borders or within the design.

I think of my daughter's grandmother-in-law, who has embarked on a series of ambitious crocheting projects as a response to her grief over her daughter's stroke. It is a way for her to move from one moment to the next, one day to the next, measuring her progress while living with a situation in which there can be none. She has made my daughter and me some beautiful shawls and complete outfits for my granddaughter's dolls, a way of giving that is no longer possible with her own daughter. While women's handwork has been traditionally viewed as a lesser pastime, or as just a pastime, it has much deeper significance.

᠅᠅᠅

A most unrealistic social view of the disabled is that we cannot experience the pleasures of the body and that having a physical limitation means that our whole selves are impaired. My friend Eva, who is blind, knows my steps and relies on sound to guide her. Anyone who has seen Evelyn Glennie, the Scottish percussionist who is deaf, leaning over her instruments and responding to them as if she and they were one understands that she is hearing with her whole body. Helen Keller, who was born deaf, mute, and blind, could smell a storm approaching, could feel the air vibrate after a flock of birds clattered off into the sky. The body has its own wisdom and continues to enjoy its many attributes even when in distress.

I can attest that my body is still a source of delight. I revel in the joys of touch, of walking down the street holding my husband's hand, of his physical presence when we are home together, or of just sitting over a long dinner.

I remember a gathering of my women's writing group some years after it had disbanded, where one of us was just recovering from a fall and another had just celebrated her 75th birthday. Our cocktails consisted of mineral water or fruit juice with only a few of us drinking alcohol. But we were each dressed to the nines and the topic of our conversation was about the pleasures of sex.

I come from a culture where people kiss one another on each cheek when they meet or leave a friend, where hugging is usual, and where my cousin and I link arms when we walk down the street. When my children were tiny, they spent much time on my lap and were lavished with hugs and kisses as they grew. When my students were bereft at some event in their lives, or feeling needy, I hugged them too. It can be the language of safety and reassurance.

When my first grandchild was born, I felt that our bodies are nothing short of a miracle, not shells but our very being. The night after our grand-daughter Ariel was born, I gathered her in my arms, feeling as if I were holding the whole world. In the months to come, I experienced the utter delight of seeing this small but very substantial person take on the world and express herself in so many ways. I listened to her chirps, applauded her early staggers as she began to walk. I watched her absorption as she took apart a toy with my daughter's long, precise fingers, as she furrowed her brow in concentration, the image of her mother. She was discovering the world with her whole body-self in continual wonder. It's as if she had given me a second life.

My little great-nephew Jae was born a month before Ariel. When he and my niece Mia returned from a few days in the hospital, I spent the most delicious morning holding him in my arms. As I spoke to him, his eyes were wide open, unusual for a newborn. I left wrapped in the presence of this new person.

I need to rest frequently when my granddaughter Ariel is visiting, and I can play for only two hours with Jae. Although I often wish I had more energy, the hours I do have are very precious to me. Mia had another little boy two years later, and I continue to enjoy their short visits when we play with the cars and trucks in our kitchen, where I keep their stash of toys. My niece is extremely sensitive to my limitations and keeps her visits short as well as cleaning up after her boys and after the simple lunch I prepare for them.

But as my granddaughter passed the toddler stage and began nursery school, she wanted trips to the museum and to the park when she and her mother came to visit, outings my body couldn't possibly support. When my daughter and my husband take off for the Boston Museum of Science for the afternoon, I can't help but feel inadequate and compare myself to my mother.

When my mother became a grandmother, she was the vice president of marketing for a firm specializing in a line of dresses she designed. She had a heavy schedule but always managed to fly in from New York City weekends to be with my children. She would arrive Friday night; Saturday morning at five o'clock they would wake her with shrieks of joy and spend the day playing with her. As they grew up, they would take the shuttle to New York City to take in the circus, the theater, and roam around the city with her.

But if I don't have physical ease I do have a feverish imagination, and this has been the bond keeping Ariel and me in our own loving world. When she comes to visit, my study floor becomes a vast housing complex with my daughter's dollhouse furniture and miniature families scattered around the room. We spend mornings with the door shut for privacy, and the scenes are more intense and vivid than *Shrek* and *Shrek 2*. I am the witch, kidnapping the children as I crow in a high-pitched voice. There are often mass kidnappings and rescues that Ariel directs. I build a jail for witches out of an old box.

Sometimes the dollhouse families need to take refuge from the marauding witch, and then we hide in the forest; I take leaves off my hibiscus plant and create a sanctuary. Or they take a slow ride down the river Seine in Paris in my slipper.

If her mother or grandfather opens the door, Ariel will say, "Mommy [or Grandpa], I love you, but will you please go away."

I bring in little scraps of my quilting material, and we create swimming pools and fields for the dolls. I bring in empty boxes for ambulances and fast cars. The hours slip by, and then invariably I have to make lunch or dinner. "Oh why do we have to eat?" Ariel protests. "I don't want to stop."

She visits once or twice a year, and those rare visits, unfortunately, are almost the only times I see her. Although my husband flies to London frequently, I can travel there only very rarely, because of my decreasing stamina. This is the one side of my life that remains a source of great frustration. I miss not only the child I utterly adore but also the very important stages in her growing and her rapid changes. The last time she left after a visit, she wrapped her arms around me as if she didn't wish to let me go. The old adages about quality time sound very good intellectually, but my arms long to hug her more often.

꙳꙳꙳

My diet may be very restricted now, but evening meals are still an important ceremony for me. Both my husband and I come from cultures where the enjoyment of preparing and sharing food is very important. When we are in France and Italy with our families, we celebrate around the table for many hours. The joy and conviviality of being with family more than compensate for my diet. It is only when we go out to restaurants that my restrictions seem to create the Great Wall of China around me as I try to explain to the puzzled waiters and waitresses the long list of foods and spices I cannot have.

But I honor my nose for filling me with such luxuries. When my husband has a particularly nice glass of wine, I inhale its odors as I once did when we were wine tasting in Burgundy many years ago. A fine wine from the Burgundy region such as an Aloxe Corton has the faint odor of raspberry beneath its earthy smell. I can tell a good wine, fruity and mellow, from a young, acidic one just by sniffing it.

Odors are stored in our memory and surface when we least expect them. I remember the time when we were first married and, although on a low budget, my husband bought a bottle of red burgundy called Pommard. I was astonished by the depth of its aroma and by its velvety texture. I also recall tasting *gentiane*, a very strong, white liqueur made from the roots of gentians, the first time we were having dinner in a tiny farm in the Alps. I felt as if I were tasting the mountain's rich soil, its meadows and wildflowers. Now, when I lean over my husband's glass of *gentiane*, I revisit that experience. He takes a sugar cube and dips it into the liqueur so the sting can be neutralized by the sugar and I can eat it. In France that is called making a "canard."

It is not only the odor of food that delights me but also of wet earth after a rain, of eucalyptus trees, of the lindens on the Paris streets that spill their fragrance on those who walk beneath them. Smells wrap us in their immediacy. When I was a very small child and my mother was at work, I used to open her closet door and hold her clothes to me just to breathe in the perfume she wore, which was such a part of her presence. Today, on the rare occasions when I run into someone who happens to be wearing Miss Dior perfume, she is suddenly before me.

I remember taking a walk in late afternoon after a day of struggling with acute pain. The world seemed to open its many corridors as I walked. There was a dense carpet of apple blossom petals on the ground, a spring snowfall of fragrance. The air was alive with birds, the lawns with colors.

I kept walking, willing myself to move, and looked up at a sky that glistened with swaths of gray, shading to more intense colors, wrapping the sun in heavy gauze. My body was still able to enjoy that exquisite spring afternoon.

When I am reconnected to nature, exploring its wonders, it is a relief from the onslaught of pressures most ill people face. Ever since my family moved from New York City to Wilmette, Illinois, when I was ten years old, I have been in love with trees. Over the years my husband and I have planted a variety of trees in our backyard, and I always gaze at their transformations through my study windows. Even in winter I love the deep blue shadows our bare pin oaks cast over the snow, losing myself in the patterns they create. My illness moves off center, and my body seems to soar and merge with the ever-changing vistas.

New England is steeped in Puritanism. Our culture is work oriented in the narrow sense, and our pleasures often artificial because they are inspired by advertisements. Imagine reading a novel in bed one morning, resting and listening to music! Or imagine just reveling in the wind flowing through the leaves in the middle of summer, feeling as if you were traveling in a river of air, or lazing in a warm ocean during the summer, riding the buoyancy of salt water.

In a cultural tradition that can be traced all the way back to the Platonic separation of reason and affect, with the latter at the very lowest level politically and philosophically, it is important to bring the body back into our conscious respect, not as an object to shape, but as a system that teaches us again and again that it cannot be conquered but must work in partnership with the will. This attitude turns our whole thinking upside down, most especially when viewed within some religious traditions. When I connect deeply with my body and feel its joy, the sense of utter powerlessness that so often assails me drains away.

10

FINDING THE LIGHT IN DARKNESS

M Y F R I E N D Sheila once told me about her sister's reaction to the radiation treatments for her cancer and about her own discouragement and exhaustion—"You go into a black hole, then you climb out and you're all right for a few days. Then it begins again"—experiences I know only too well when I seem caught in a period when I am unable to do much and feel imprisoned by my physical frailty.

Black holes are part of my life. But it is strange how those of us who are seriously ill can live a duality: a daily grind of relentless suffering on the one hand and illuminations on the other, blessings that come when I least expect them.

Since 2001 I have been absent from myself because of chronic insomnia, partly resulting from the sleep disturbances accompanying fibromyalagia. As I am someone who typically needs many hours of sleep at night, albeit interrupted, plus a two-hour nap, this is torture. Being absent from myself means I cannot participate fully in events at the Women's Studies Research Center; means not being able to go to the artists' retreat where I traditionally work on my poetry; means I lack energy even to write in my journal; means not going out to visit friends, or to a museum or a concert—everything that nourishes my soul. In effect, living with four hours of sleep at night means living in isolation and with a frozen mind, the days blurring past without markings. It also means that I grumble to myself continually how weary I am of living.

However, I am visited again and again by reminders that I am accompanied on this difficult journey, reminders that appear like butterflies flickering in the depth of a forest. Were I not in such a dark and seemingly hopeless situation, I would not notice those fragile wings swooping over me again and again. Nor would I be rereading the poems of the thirteenth-century religious scholar and Sufi mystic Rumi with an understanding that radiates throughout my being. "Darkness is your candle./ Your boundaries are your quest./ You must have shadow and light source both./ Listen, and lay down your head under the tree of awe."[1]

These flickering visitations take many forms. Among the most surprising are letters from people I barely know. In August 2003 I gave a presentation at a book club my husband and I belong to. I must admit I had to exercise all my powers of persuasion to have the members read *Song of the Exile*,[2] a searing account of the Chinese and Korean "comfort women" enslaved by the Japanese army during World War II, a historical episode that has been shrouded in silence. The club members were understandably reluctant because they see their reading as a form of entertainment and a relief from the pressures of work. I prevailed and gave a presentation about the way women and girls as young as twelve were dragged from schools and, for the duration of the war, were subjected to multiple rapes daily, with the vast majority dying from abuse and malnutrition. Discussion was brisk even though, by the fixed smiles of a number of people, I knew not everyone had read the book.

That was the last book club meeting I was able to attend, so I was surprised when, in mid-December, I received a note from a member I knew only slightly. That letter arrived at a time when my day's accomplishments were limited to small household chores and reading. Such a schedule was a painful contrast to the two or three hours of intense working time I had once had, making me feel utterly useless. I tucked the card into my journal, savoring its kind message: "*Song of the Exile* was a gift from all that you are. Your intellectual and artistic achievements are a candle in the dark," and at the end of her card she wrote, "Your health, I realize, remains fragile. How all of us wish it were not so. My thoughts are with you in encouragement and emotional sustenance, Tenderly Lillian." That comment moved me deeply, for my trials are invisible to most people.

The following week I received an e-mail from the author of *Song of the Exile*, the Hawaiian writer Kiana Davenport. We had never met, but I had written to her two years earlier when I first read her book, and we had exchanged letters. In September I sent her a copy of my latest book

---

1. C. Barks with J. Moyne, *The Essential Rumi* (HarperSanFrancisco, 1996), 20. The quoted passages are from the poem "Enough Words?"
2. K. Davenport, *Song of the Exile* (Random House, New York, 1999).

of poems. The week I heard from her, I was in one of the periodic moods of intense self-doubt that many writers are prone to, which was deepened by the fact that I hadn't written poetry in so many months. I'm a third-rate poet, I kept thinking to myself, out of sync with contemporary interests, irrelevant. Kiana's e-mail was the most wonderful gift: "Mahalo, thank you a million times for *Wind, Frost and Fire*. It is beautiful. The imagery is stunning. I have read it over and over. I love good poetry, and yours is exceptional, sweeping across different countries, aware of the ravages wrought out in the world as I hope I do. So many poets and novelists write tight little books that seem to be so myopic, I cannot grasp them." That note made me remember the comment the Nobel Prize–winning poet Joseph Brodsky made to a news anchorman when he was asked, "How many people do you feel you need to compose a good audience?" "Three," he answered to the anchorman's utter surprise.

Yet another letter came in the same week, this time with a photo and a Christmas card. The previous July, the cousin of a Mexican friend had come to Boston with her little daughter, who needed heart surgery. I wrote to the little girl, Ybi, sending her the pop-up cards children love and telling her she had a grandmother in the United States. And then, since the operation was a success, Ybi became a distant memory. But her parents wrote me a long letter including a beautiful photo of five-year-old Ybi with long, black hair and an enchanting, mischievous smile. On the back her mother wrote, "With much affection to my grandmother, Marguerite whom I will always remember as someone special in my life." Her mother's note spoke of the loneliness of sitting on the seventeenth floor of the Massachusetts General Hospital in an alien country surrounded by a strange language and of how my cards had given her solace. She told me that they had seemed like an answer to her need for accompaniment.

These three events happening within such a short time made me reflect that there is another level of awareness we pass by in our hurried lives, a level that knows no time or geography and where we are instruments of consolation, speaking to each other in the secret recesses of our beings. In his beautiful and strange poem "Birdsong from inside the Egg," Rumi wrote, "Then . . . God bends and whispers . . . 'Beggar, spread out / your robe. I'll fill it with gold. / I've come to protect your consciousness. / Where has it gone? Come back into awareness!'"[3]

---

3. Barks, *The Essential Rumi*, 274.

I was also awakened to the recognition of God's grace by unexpected kind gestures. The night the United States invaded Iraq with a strategy of "shock and awe" I was moderating a panel at Brandeis on women and spirituality, to celebrate our diversity and common humanity. In a room above the student union, the rector at St. John's Episcopal Church in Jamaica Plain; the founder and director of the Mistabra Institute of Jewish Textual Activism; a spiritual leader of the Wompanoag Nation; and Humaira Kirmani, who is active in the Wayland Mosque, countered with presentations of wisdom and reverence. Humaira and I felt an instant kinship. When we had lunch a few months later we were able to speak from the heart about my daughter's and her daughter's illnesses and how concerned we were, a subject that haunts me and that I rarely discuss outside the family.

A year passed before we met again. This too was in mid-December, when I could only spend time with people who understood that an hour was all the time I could manage with a friend. "How are you? You look tired," Humaira commented, whereas most people say, "Oh, you look wonderful." Humaira went right to the heart of our concerns as we spoke of our daughters again and of those difficult times. I shared a very strange experience I had had many years ago and that I had never spoken of, telling her about my visit to an exhibit of Turkish miniatures at Harvard's Sackler Museum. I paused in front of a panel of black Arabic letters that sent waves of emotion through me. "God," I whispered to myself, and indeed, when I looked at the translation below, I saw the word *Allah*. Rather than trying to deny my experience, Humaira merely smiled and commented, "You are open."

In that one hour, Humaira told me about the chilling fear enveloping her community as a result of repeated calls from and interrogations by the FBI, and about banks suddenly closing her people's accounts. I understood, for my family had fled to the United States to escape fascism in Italy during World War II. We shared each other's experiences, reaching across the barriers of culture, history, and language, two women in a small corner of the world, holding it together amid so much hatred. Such instances of peace may be quiet and unnoticed by the world, but they are important. Interwoven in our discussion was Humaira's gift of understanding and of the faith that kept her at her prayers every afternoon. A few days later she called me: "Marguerite, I am sending you a prayer my husband translated for you. Keep it under your pillow. It will help you sleep."

And as if these blessings were not enough, I recently experienced the miracle of turkey soup and my niece's love during a difficult time when my husband was out of the country. My niece was so busy with her active little boys, only two years apart, that I could barely have a conversation with her over the telephone much less when the three of them were with me. But during that visit, my quiet niece took one look at me and said, "I am going to make you some turkey soup so you won't have to cook this week." Despite the fact that she lived an hour's drive away and that she needed to chauffeur her children to nursery school, she showed up at my door the following day with a large container of soup. The next week she arrived with a vegetable casserole. This was a big commitment for a mother whose days were endless and whose nights were often punctuated by one of her boys wandering into her and her husband's room. This too was a wonderful expression of love. My niece, who is often uncomfortable verbalizing her feelings, spoke through turkey soup and a casserole.

What illness has taught me is that experiences that may appear inconsequential in the rush of everyday life can have both spaciousness and a resonance. And sometimes, events that may at first seem disconnected make a whole if we are truly open. For me, this gathering of discontinuities is the closest I can come to meaning during my dark periods. Ironically, it is when I am unable to do more than struggle through the day that I seem to see with a new depth and to understand that the wounds life inflicts are what open us to these insights. As Rumi wrote, "The grief you cry out from / draws you toward union. / Your pure sadness / that wants help / is the secret cup."[4]

The journal I keep on the night table beside my bed may be full of gaps from the many months when I couldn't even write a few sentences, but now it is bulging with the cards and messages I have received. That they came within such a short period and at a time when I was so discouraged helped me realize that I am neither invisible nor alone.

I know now, even though days may pass when I seem to be walking in utter darkness, that God is speaking to me with many voices. When I keep asking myself "Why, why do I have to suffer so stupidly, relentlessly, and invisibly?" these replies arrive like the glittering wings of the Monarch butterflies I have so often admired. My questioning, my discouragement,

---

4. Ibid., 155, 156. The quoted passage is from the poem "Love Dogs."

and these responses are part of an ongoing and strange conversation of the heart. Rumi captured it in his line from the poem "A Basket of Fresh Bread": "Stay bewildered in God."[5]

᠊ᢧᢧᢧ᠊

We think of medicine as responding to physical symptoms and expect much of the medical profession, as did I when I first became ill. But the body in pain affects the psyche, the heart, and the spirit. While speaking with a therapist may have helped me face the emotional burdens of my condition in the early years, I discovered that it was above all my spirit that needed attention and that by drawing on pastimes that gave me pleasure I could regenerate my thirst for life. I remember my high school English teacher telling our soporific class on Shakespeare that reading his work was important and that "someday it will open a window." I didn't know what she meant at the time, but I sensed the importance of what she said, and it stayed with me; often as adults we need to soar beyond our circumstances to find ourselves. The window through literature, art, and music connects me to the world in new and profound ways. It not only serves as an outlet for the turbulence of my feelings; it gives me a spaciousness that contrasts with my disabilities.

It was my mother who made certain that I was exposed to all three art forms from a very early age. Even when we were just making ends meet, my mother always provided me with books, fairy tales from around the world and then serious literature. From the time I could read, I spent many hours curled up in a quiet corner with my favorite book, transported to a world beyond our apartment.

She also brought me to concerts and to the opera as a special treat when I became an adolescent, and I can still remember watching the famous conductor Toscanini as he brought to life Debussy's *La Mer*. My mother was wise enough to expose me to this world before I was drawn to the usual teen tastes.

Music is medicine for the whole body. I always remember the calming effect of the New Age tapes my daughter sent me during the early years of my illness, and how they accompanied me during so many nights. The priest I met at the conference of hospice workers in Longwood, California, where I was a speaker told me how he would pipe in New Age music

---

5. Ibid., 256.

to comfort the dying. When my niece Michele's husband was preparing to have an operation for the removal of a cancerous kidney, she arranged with his surgeon to have a CD of Mozart playing during the procedure, believing that this would both accompany him and help the procedure go smoothly, which is exactly what happened.

Sacred music has always inspired me, and even though I am no longer a practicing Catholic I love sitting in churches and listening to choirs, especially to Gregorian chants. They give me a feeling of metaphysical order and comfort. When we are in France, my husband and I always drive to St. Bernard Pass in the Alps where the ancient abbey that once served as a refuge is still perched on the side of a high peak. I like to sit in the small chapel and listen to the singing of the mass, feeling the music flow through my whole being, giving it wings.

There are times when my grief over my condition needs an echo, and then I turn to Henryk Górecki or Arvo Pärt, for East European composers have a particular genius for combining tragedy with transcendence, as their peoples have over centuries. Their works are powerful without being heavy and have the sweep of an ocean and a sobriety of tone that have accompanied me over and over again. I have lent these CDs to friends who have experienced loss, and they have found comfort in being in-cluded in a wider circle of sorrow expressed with such beauty. Music sweeps us into another universe where our sadness finds expression, yet moves off center into the contemplation of the energy and spirit that pervades us all.

Such an obvious remedy—and yet it never occurred to me as a way of healing until desperation urged me on, as if I had just thought of hiking shoes to make a difficult climb easier.

What also helps me rise above the daily torments of unpredictable pain and insomnia is perusing my collection of art books and going to art exhibits when possible. My mother started bringing me to art museums when I was five years old. I vividly remember my very first visit, standing transfixed in front of a single sunflower by Vincent van Gogh that had so much vibrancy it seemed to be exploding from the frame. Gazing at that sunflower was the beginning of a lifelong interest in and love of art that led me to study art history in college and, with my mother's help, assemble a collection of books on the subject over the years.

Because she worked long hours, my mother always made certain I would be occupied during her absence. I attended art classes, learning to block-print and silk-screen. At one point I had a kiln in my bedroom, where I made jewelry and small objects as the burn marks on the rug proliferated. I now realize why my mother wanted me to learn how to use my hands and to create beauty. It was a pastime that would ferry me through dark waters.

When I began writing poetry, I realized that art is intimately connected to my writing, for my poems are very visual and filled with images. Art is yet another way of seeing with the whole self and an inspiration that often sparks new poems. I not only write poems that were sparked by paintings but also consider paintings yet another form of poetry. As a poet I think analogically; one image calls up another event or image. Like painters, I put together disparate insights, or take the chaos we live in and try to create order.

In the crush of my very busy life as a professor, parent, and volunteer, I rarely had time to pursue this interest. Since each hour was accounted for in my long days, the art books stayed unopened, and I was able to see only a few of the unusual exhibits that came to the Boston Museum of Fine Arts. The ones I did manage to attend were memorable, but my response to them was very different from the way I now enter the world of painting.

Going to an art exhibit is always an exhilarating experience for me, even though I tire easily and have such difficulty standing that I can stay at most thirty minutes, with frequent breaks for sitting down. Still, these visits are exceedingly precious. I am communicating across time, from soul to soul. Most important, my family has given me catalogues of these exhibits as gifts, and I keep a number of them in my bedroom to carry me through difficult times.

Over the years, I have become increasingly drawn to artists who have movement, passion, and tumult in their work. One Sunday, while visiting my son Pierre in New York City, I lured both him and my husband to an exhibit of the French expressionist painter Chaim Soutine at the Jewish Museum. His canvases were flickering with color, movement, and light. A still life with fish glowed with orange flashes, a forest in Ausieres made the wind visible as the trees bent under its weight and seemed to be traveling in place at great speed. One particular painting of a small town in Provence struck me with its river of blues, greens, and yellows as if the town were poured into my senses in one gulp. All of Soutine's works seemed swept by gales of emotion. It was as if I were looking into the mirror of my own heart, at the tempests that are invisible to most people: they are seemingly chaotic, but with the order that vision and suffering imposes.

An artist friend who attended the same exhibit told me that she had to leave after a few moments because she found it too overwhelming and the colors overly intense. But I found an affirmation of my inner life.

Although I love revisiting my favorite artists, I am happiest when discovering work that exposes me to different cultures. Once, before I became ill and while I accompanied my husband on a business trip to Sidney, Australia, I visited an exhibit of aboriginal art in the Sidney Art Museum. I was both perplexed and deeply moved by the swirls of multicolored dots that seemed as if they were both static and in motion. Although I knew little about the history of these people, I somehow felt I was in the presence of deeply spiritual work. But it was only in 2000, when we attended a more extensive exhibit, that I persisted in spending as much time as possible before those paintings. Fortunately there were explanatory paragraphs beside each painting and benches where I could rest while studying them. As I sat there lost in my own thoughts, I began to see that the paintings were in effect journeys of different kinds—in search of a partner, in search of a water hole—and that they were depicting sacred rituals that were interwoven with everyday life as well as with the ongoing creation of this earth.

I was struck by the similarity of some of the colors to the unusual palette of Hopi art. I remember visiting a now abandoned kiva in Arizona many years ago and being drawn by the dream images moving through the circular structure, which were rendered in lavenders, pale oranges, rose, and soft yellows, combinations of colors I experienced as a lost language.

One of the most surprising discoveries I made recently was before a vast collection of ancient Chinese calligraphy at a special exhibit in the Metropolitan Museum in New York City. I didn't know what to expect and was stunned by the great differences in personality I could detect among the calligraphers as I walked through room after room of huge scrolls. I discovered that some were poems and paused in front of a thirteenth-century text that seemed to come out of my own experience: "Brush and ink are my hoe and plow / no ditches furrow my remote spirit / no boundaries limit my mind." I found myself drawn into a silent conversation with the personalities expressed in the calligraphers' brushstrokes.

As always, such moments inspired me to educate myself, and that too has been another kind of journey. As a result, when I enter a really difficult period, I can stretch out on my bed with catalogues from exhibits and journey to the outback of Australia or to ancient China, where calligraphy was the ultimate visual expression.

I used this dark time of insomnia to study the aesthetics and history of Chinese calligraphy. I learned about the different script styles and how these are intended to convey different moods to the viewer, for example the calm detachment of the sutra texts, written in orderly standard script, or the restless agitation of the wild cursive style.

Oddly, just when I was feeling that my daily life was being fragmented, I experienced a deep continuity on another level, for I discovered that the calligraphy I was so absorbed in is a form of body language. In some texts the calligrapher's inner states of elation, anger, or grief are revealed in characters that lose the vertical and horizontal axes governing the placement of strokes, or even fuse. In a general's eulogy for a son killed in battle, the strokes are a nearly illegible tangle of characters, of twisting and jabbing attacks on the paper. Interestingly, Chinese scholars typically refer to characters as having muscle, bone, and flesh, as expressing pent-up rage or bone-deep pain. As I pored over my books, I saw my own story written there.

ᴥ ᴥ ᴥ

It was my sleepless nights and feelings of despair, plus a very small book with pages of handmade mulberry-leaf paper my daughter once gave me, that started me writing psalms. I had left the book untouched for many years, thinking it was too precious to mar with writing, for the pages had a beautiful texture and were a pleasure just to hold. Then, when I went through this insomniac period, I found myself writing down my thoughts, not in an orderly fashion, but haphazardly during the night or before turning out the light. As the months passed, I shaped them into prayers and began a book. As the prayers came tumbling out, I found that they gathered all that I had learned during my long journey, including my feelings of deep connection with this troubled world.

For instance, one night I was quietly watching the moon through the slats on our bedroom window when this prayer came tumbling out:

MINDFULNESS

May I not be caught
in the turbulence of my days,
but awaken to the moon glowing
through branches, tufts

ᔊ 121 ᔊ

of new grass among
melting snow.
May I always remain
a child, drawn
by wonder at what is.[6]

In times of stress, such as the tunnels I experience, ordinary events and
sights can suddenly flare like lit matches. They are like the unexpected
kind gestures that ferry me through the waters of night. I carry these flares
in my head for days on end, and they reappear in that small book with
mulberry-leaf paper that is on my nightstand. One gray April morning,
the sight of green tendrils on the pin oak outside my study window awakened something deep within me and sparked yet another prayer.

THE HOLY BOOK

It is the doorway
into our beginnings,
the cloud of feathery
green shoots rising
from that cosmic tree.
Humility is written there
and grandeur.
Our seeing deeply
into all that surrounds us,
our awakening, all inscribed
in the body's sacred text.[7]

I wanted to put the human body back into the center of spirituality,
removing the sting of shame that accompanies it in so many interpreta-
tions of traditional religions and also in society.

PRAISE THE WOUNDED

Praise the child
in the wheelchair
for he is whole.

---

6. M. Bouvard, *Prayers for Comfort in Difficult Times* (Wind Publications, Nicholas-
ville, Kentucky, 2004), 32.
7. Ibid., 55.

> Praise the blind man
> for he sees
> in a different way.
> Praise the deaf woman
> who hears
> with all of her body
> and the person who is deaf
> and blind for she can feel
> the air vibrate long
> after the swans have flown.[8]

It was not only seemingly everyday sights that inspired me but also the waves of extraordinary events lapping around me, which resonated even more deeply because of the tormented period I was traversing. For instance, late one night I heard an ambulance pulling up in front of my neighbor's house. She and I were very close, and I knew that her husband, who was ill with cancer, was having a crisis. I put a coat over my robe and rushed across the street. In fact her husband was dying, was coughing up blood. I put my arms around my friend and held her close while she screamed, "He's never coming back, he's never coming back," as the ambulance drove away. The following week I wrote this prayer for her as a gift, and she put it in a frame on her dresser.

GRIEF

> Dear God, the death
> of my loved one
> has left me broken
> and rudderless with empty days
> stretching before me.
> Lead me out of silence towards a new path,
> heal the anguish
> in my heart,
> make me whole again.[9]

Late at night, as I scribbled my often disconnected thoughts across the pages of that small book, those notes not only became a new book; they

---

8. Ibid., 76.
9. Ibid., 24.

bore me across the darkness. I remembered one of my favorite works, written by the editor of the French magazine *Elle*, Jean-Dominque Bauby, who had suffered a stroke. He was almost totally paralyzed and could no longer speak, but he had developed an alphabet that he could convey by the way he blinked his eyes. Slowly and painfully, he wrote a short book about his illness that became a best seller.

And thus I ended my book of prayers:

QUESTIONS

When a flash flood of tears
sweeps over my borders
and I shake my fist at the empty air
You remind me how music is born.

When I question the history books,
the phalanxes of raw recruits
torn from their mothers' arms
You answer I am a minnow
trying to chart the ocean.[10]

10. Ibid., 64.

11

BLESSINGS

WHILE THE environment may be one of the many complex elements causing my physical problems, illness has raised the larger question of meaning for me. In the early years, I framed that question as why me? with considerable anguish. Since then, my attitude has shifted, and I think why not me? I look around and see many who are worse off than I am, see that suffering is part of our story and that eventually the great majority of people become marked by tragedy in some way. This lesson was before me in my grandmother's and mother's lives and losses, although when I was young, I foolishly believed I was somehow exempt because my immediate family had escaped the ravages of World War II and because I always enjoyed good health.

The most important avenue to gaining a perspective on my illness has been my practice of meditation. It makes me realize how lucky I am because I think of so many people tangled in war and violence, of Honduras and El Salvador in the aftermath of terrible storms and flooding. Although I grumble about having to spend so much time in doctors' offices, I realize how fortunate I am to have access to medical care and to have a roof over my head. And though this illness has made my body prematurely old in the sense of all the limitations it imposes on my life, I am indeed lucky to have been able to have the career I worked for, to have been able to support my children in so many ways. I think of all the ill youngsters who have never had a chance to pass unencumbered through life's stages. And I remember my dear friend Ana's reply to me when I expressed surprise that she sends so much of her small income to her relatives in Cuba. She looked at me and said, "At least I eat every day!"

As the years passed, I realized I was doing not only some self-examination but also some deep observation of all the people in my life. I have come to know myself in a different way, and that helps me appreciate how someone else may see things differently than I do, how that has come to be. Deep meditation is an act of inclusion. When I enter myself, I see everyone, not in relation to me, but in relation to his or her own self, history, and situation. Meditation then is not a passive experience but a very active one of reflection.

When I am in the mountains or walking in the woods surrounding the small lake in our town, I lose myself in the reflection of water against a tree trunk, the scent and feel of pine needles beneath my feet. This too is a form of meditation, a form of seeing with the whole body-mind/heart.

I have created a way of living with my many obstacles by working on my inner space in a society that measures by externals. This has taught me to draw on my own resources, to recognize that I have them, to travel to periods of my childhood when I had significant learning experiences. This is where I bring my ongoing inner conversations about meaning, where I reconnect with a faith that too often slips away when I am experiencing a particularly trying episode. In that sense it is an utterly free zone in which I allow all those emotions such as rage, sadness, and despair condemned by both religion and society.

While in parochial school as a young child, I was repeatedly told that despair was a terrible sin. However, I have found that plunging down and regrouping is part of the journey through a chronic condition, the zigzagging trail of the spirit that is always with me. When I speak with friends who have suffered loss, I realize that this is not unusual and that living with authenticity means embracing rather than denying the harsh terms of our existence. Only then can we begin to transcend such conditions.

When I pause at the end of the day and question the universe, I sometimes get answers in my head, not complete answers, but the fragment of a thought that points me in a different direction. For example, once when I was still struggling with the newness of fibromyalgia, I found myself feeling I was worthless. Then the thought arose, No one who loves is ever worthless. Another time, I was lamenting my many physical limitations when the phrase "You have everything you need in your heart" suddenly appeared in my thoughts. Part of meditation has become a dialogue between the perplexity that continually arises as a result of living so close to the edge and the responses that come tumbling into my head when I least expect them.

I have come to experience meditation as a prayerful way of life, as learning to see more deeply and clearly, as traveling beyond our separateness, for it has strengthened my passionate engagement with the outside world. I connect with my breathing and my beating heart, intent on that source of life energy which is always there, waiting for me to acknowledge it, to drink from its well.

One night, while I was browsing through a book of Australian aboriginal myths and paintings, a paragraph leapt out at me. It dealt with the initiation of the young into adulthood: "in an aura of mystery, the initiate endures ordeals of pain and trials of fortitude whose significance remains with him the rest of his life," and "these initiation rituals may extend over many years."[1]

In many branches of the Christian faith, believers look to the afterlife as compensation for our trials on this earth, and some religions stress reincarnation as the explanation for harsh circumstances. The Australian aborigines, who represent one of the oldest civilizations, believe suffering is part of our journey and we must learn to live with it, not as an aberration, but as part of an ongoing education through which we grow in strength and endurance. These wise people do not grapple with the question of why we suffer, which assails us continually in a society that seems to worship "happiness" or "success," whatever those states are supposed to mean. They understand that trying circumstances are a part of life.

⟡⟡⟡

We live in a multicultural society, and if we have learned anything from our diversity, it is that truths are as various as our religions and lifestyles. If we are freed from the eternal question of *why*, so that we no longer feel singled out, we can then address the most important task of *how*: how to respond to illness. Chronic illness has given me the opportunity to reassess my life, to decide on how I will live, what I hope to accomplish, and what is important to me. As a writer on medical ethics, Arthur Frank, pointed out, illness is a moral occasion: it raises for each one of us the question of who we are, who we will become. It raises the question of how we will use the time and energy that remains. What may have been important when we enjoyed good health may now seem insignificant. Some people may change as a result of their situation and others become more of who they were.

While we all wrestle with moral choices in our working and private

---

1. C. P. Mountford, *The Dreamtime Book: Australian Aboriginal Myths* (Prentice-Hall, Englewood Cliff, New Jersey, 1973), 11.

lives, illness makes the question of choice more urgent. Given the severe limitations I experience in arranging my time, I want to spend it in a worthwhile way. Like many of the disabled, who are regarded as less valuable by society, I want very much to be of use. Ironically, grappling with my various conditions has given me qualities that have proved socially valuable, most particularly a deeper understanding of and compassion for others. My own pain has taught me how to accompany people in distress.

A colleague of mine in political science quit her teaching job after a long episode with cancer and decided to spend her time in public service, organizing and heading a political research center. For some of us who are ill, a new sensitivity to our connections with the world inspires us to want to give in new ways, to make our lives more meaningful.

I have also gained a more profound appreciation of the struggles of other people and a new perspective on what really constitutes a good and satisfying life. Of this I am sure: if I could regain my health, I would never again return to my former hurried pace or to what once seemed so important to me. My friend Vera, who survived Auschwitz, wrote that she no longer worried about lost keys or dust accumulating on the furniture but had learned how to treasure life because of what she had experienced in that hell.

It is ironic that being faced with a distressed body and with my own helplessness has brought me to a new level of awareness. I have learned that moments of illumination or serenity are interwoven with dark times, are two sides of the same coin, and that I can live with one side of me in the Arctic and the other in the tropics. This new awakening has made me feel a tremendous gratitude for my life and all it holds. I often quietly express praise throughout the day, not just during religious ceremonies or meditation.

My growing spirituality has also given me a new attitude toward death. It is something I ponder often while I am meditating. However, it has become a friend, exhorting me to use each moment well, rather than a feared enemy. Now I am aware of it, not in a morbid way, but as another step in the journey of life and the soul.

One of the most important lessons I have learned is that it is attitude, not circumstances, that matters. Perhaps the gold at the end of the rainbow is the wisdom, understanding, acceptance, and fortitude so prized by the Australian aborigines, the ability to be fully awake to life's possibilities, to mine my inner self as well as my surroundings. No one will cheer me for developing these abilities, for they have not earned social esteem, but these abilities promote what cosmologists call, when they refer to the catastrophic explosion of supernovas, the "lushness of regeneration." I am not passive in the unending creation but, like so many of my ill friends, a participator and an unsung activist.

My friend Eva is a shining example of how someone who is ill has grown as a result of her condition. She may be blind and fettered by a most painful rheumatoid arthritis, but she has learned many languages, including Russian, French, German, and a smattering of Chinese, so that she is at home throughout the world. She may be blind, but she has a Harvard doctorate in human rights law as well as two OBEs (Order of the British Empire award), which she laughingly tells me are too large to wear.

It is not just understanding but, more important, a love of life that fuels her and me, and so many ill people. That passion need not be grandiose. Comparisons between our efforts are not useful, and one person's accomplishments are not necessarily more significant than another person's just because they happen to be public and wide ranging.

I see my life journey as one of continual transformations. While these include loss with its attendant pain, they are also an important part of my growth. For instance, when each of my children became an adult, I lost a child but gained a friend, and the satisfaction of seeing the completion of my efforts, and the unfolding of a substantial person I continually discover.

Because of the many changes resulting from my illnesses, my life is now so different from the one I once had that I could hardly have predicted it, but it is a life I cherish and am proud of, although I realize how relative that perception may be. I recently spent an hour on the telephone speaking to a young woman newly diagnosed with a very painful case of IC. I listened to her rage and despair, and at the end I described to her how I had rebuilt my own life. "Pardon me, but I think you have an awful life!" she replied. Sixteen years ago, I would have agreed. But since then, I have come to a clearer vision of who I am, and I would not describe my illness as a defining trait. It is a painful circumstance. At some point in our lives, most of us find ourselves in what may seem like unbearable situations. They are also opportunities.

Ultimately, pain and loss have given me authenticity. I feel that I have joined not only the circle of humanity but also all of nature as I sought to plumb the meaning of suffering and as my aching heart and body have come to respect their utter wholeness. I had to change my suppositions and my frame of reference. It was like being jolted awake from a dream.

꙳꙳꙳

Once, when I was seven years old and my mother and I were walking down the crowded streets of downtown New York, she stopped short in front of a store window. Because I was wrapped in my own thoughts as usual, I didn't really pay attention to what she was staring at. But since she stayed there without moving, I finally asked her what was holding her. "That's my father's silver tea set with our family initials," she said, pointing to a gleam in the window. I couldn't make a connection between those objects and our everyday lives. Nor could I put them in the context of a war I had been exposed to by a movie my mother had taken me to see and by letters from Trieste that sent her into tears. I knew nothing then about the way all sides in this terrible conflict had plundered. What I saw at that moment was her strange sadness. I asked her tentatively, "Do you think we could buy it?" "Impossible," my mother replied. I pondered this for a while, and then she turned to me with a very serious face, telling me, "We are lucky. We are alive."

As with so many things my mother told me when I was young, I had no frame of reference. But since she was not given to talking much and since she treated me as an adult when she did have something important to share, that comment was stored in my subconscious until I began to revise my values during my trek through illness. When I take stock of these difficult years of revision, I am reminded of what it feels like to see more clearly—when my glasses clear the blur of my astigmatism. It's as if my illness represents another opportunity to see my own life and the lives of those around me more completely. That new perspective has helped me reassess my values in a number of ways.

Most particularly, I have gained a deeper understanding of time. In the early years of my illness, I mourned the loss of my ability to have a schedule, to plan my days, weeks, and months. I felt as if the time available to me was steadily shrinking along with my life. Since then, I have acquired an entirely new outlook, learning how to become flexible so that I could enjoy an hour or two when it suddenly became available because I felt rested. I have learned how to prioritize and lop off superfluous activities, how to focus, and how to enjoy periods when I am unable to work as opportunities for deep thinking.

When I was a professor, I was always making lists, always rushing around with my attention wandering to the next task. Now I am focused on the present and have found the here and now full of opportunities and discoveries. When I am in a physician's waiting room, a frequent occurrence, I observe the people around me, imagining their stories, or I knit blankets for my grandchildren, or read all the material I don't have time for. Sitting in a crowded waiting room, I can read about the conflict in Macedonia, or the controversies over the genetic modification of food, or the recent elections in Italy. Even while I am on the examining table waiting for the numbing jelly to take hold before the instillation of Cystistat, I continue reading.

If I am in a trying situation either in a physician's office or while traveling, for instance, I simply go into meditation to find that inner core of calm and balance. When I must rush about to prepare for a trip, or because I have a backlog of chores, I feel extremely uncomfortable, as if I were half awake or half alive. A return to stillness, such as simply gazing out my study window at the colors and grace of the Japanese maple, always regenerates me.

One cold and windy March, I rented a small apartment on the ocean in Provincetown because I was too ill to make my scheduled trip to a writers' retreat. I needed to be by myself to face my vulnerabilities, my grief, and my feeling of powerlessness, trusting that renewal would follow as I moved through these emotions.

Every day, I strolled at my own slow pace through the narrow streets, observing the routines of the town: high school youngsters tumbling out of school, the elderly sitting on benches and chatting, mothers with strollers. As the days slipped by, the wind, the ocean, and the privacy of a small-town resort out of season took hold. I breathed in the presence of the water with its moods and shifting hues. I listened to the rustle and slap of wavelets as the tide came swishing in and gazed at the pilings wavering in sun-struck water from the window of my small apartment and indeed, by the end of a long week, regained my serenity.

I have discovered that when moments are deeply lived, they have the quality of eternity. One chilly June morning after a crowded and harried flight from Boston to Geneva, my husband and I woke up in our mountain retreat to perfect silence and open time. My body told me to nap for a few hours late morning and then early afternoon. It was five o'clock before we set off for our drive to our favorite mountain pass about an hour away, but late afternoon has always been my favorite time. The slopes were rinsed with bronze light, and there was a somnolence in the air. We slipped into the rhythm of haying time when the scent of newly mown grass drenched us and the mowing machines hummed like distant bees.

When we arrived at the mountain pass, we ambled through a meadow where cows were beginning to file down for the evening milking and the slopes echoed with the delicate timbre of their bells. The evening light moved through the mouths of buttercups, gentians, and daisies. Everything around us was breathing: the wind in my hair, the heavy snuffing of cows, the tall grasses rustling.

At a bend in the trail we sat on a ridge between two valleys, mere specks absorbed by the grandeur around us. Although there were still swaths of snow on the highest peaks, the summer pastures below us shone with the vibrancy of new growth. We saw that we could find refuge in all that will continue when we are even beyond memory and that everything surrounding us seemed be an intimation of a life that is so much greater than this one.

᚛ ᚛ ᚛

Over the years, I have developed an uncanny ability to make a day of an hour, to accomplish much without having extended periods to work. It has come through my practice of being present in my work, of being able to concentrate, not in a planned way, but whenever the moment occurs. I have discovered that it is not the length of time I spend, or its predictability, but the richness and fullness of it that matter.

There is something liberating in the seeming chaos of my days. Open time is when I am not planning, when my thoughts are free to roam, when I am not trying to direct them. It is the opposite of control. From my years of writing poetry, I know that I cannot will myself into creativity but must allow it to happen while seemingly daydreaming or performing mundane chores. In fact, during a recent period when I was unable to do much but rest in bed, I began a new project, a book about collaborative mothering. I am comfortable with the fact that such projects will unfold in due time and that I cannot begin to guess when they will reach completion. If nothing else, I have learned to respond head-on to whatever happens with my body and make the most of it.

Although I rarely have the stamina for socializing, the three friends I meet are very close to me, and it always seems as if we have just seen each other yesterday despite the long intervals separating these get-togethers. I no longer spend time on the telephone with friends. The telephone is for my adult children and their spouses and for my nieces. I no longer go shopping or visit friends except for the occasional treat of browsing in a bookstore. Even though the Women's Studies scholars have a new building to house their activities, providing work space and allowing the scholars to meet informally in the kitchen for coffee and conversation, my visits to the center are carefully spaced. I will go for seminars or for the meetings of my research group, but I cannot spend afternoons just "hanging out." However, these changes have not made me feel impoverished. I may occasionally feel wistful about wanting to have the opportunity for informal conversations with my colleagues, but I think of the way I use the hours available to me as fine-tuning my life, as honing down so that what I have vibrates with meaning.

The world-renowned astrophysicist Stephen Hawking, who can communicate only through a voice-activated computer, once remarked that his illness gave him the time to think. What he meant was that it liberated him from many social obligations aside from his family and colleagues. Thus he has had endless opportunities to ponder the cosmos and to solve problems. The terms and conditions of my life have imposed a similar solitude. However, that has meant being available to myself and having time for contemplation. I am taking the opportunity to know myself, and this has deepened my appreciation of life. I realize how much I have taken for granted over the years and have learned how to cherish what I have rather than railing at what is missing. I have come to see life as a great gift and not as a given, have learned to savor a beautiful day, a kind gesture from a friend, the utter miracle of feeling well and alert for a few hours.

Now that I no longer rush around, I look around me with wonder and praise—at people I may pass in the street, at the most minute changes that herald the seasons, at the sense of completion I feel when I think of my children and my nieces. I have come to realize that it takes a reflective way of being to become content and to feel at peace.

This unexpected opportunity has brought me to a new place. More than ever, I have a new appreciation of the depth of ordinary life. Ironically, this is a lesson I kept repeating to my students who were learning to write poetry. "Don't strive for the grandiose," I told them, "but begin with yourselves and your own experiences; they are precious." When my husband and I take one of our slow walks around Lake Waban, I always see something new that fills me with awe regardless of how many times we have circled the lake. I will marvel over the lichen on a pine tree, the pale shoots of new trees. Over the years the population of our town has changed, and I love listening to the new languages floating by as other hikers pass us talking in Russian or Chinese.

I think of my son-in-law's eighty-seven-year-old grandmother Maud, who finds joy in receiving a card from abroad, in the handwork she does, in the visits from her grandchildren, or in an afternoon out with my daughter, Laurence. She takes great pleasure in her life despite problems with her vision, her deafness, and the difficulties she has walking. There is a sign she has pasted on her refrigerator that captures her spirit: "Just do it," a phrase she lived by long before it became a marketing slogan.

One of the ordinary pleasures I experience is speaking with people whom I happen to meet during my long waits in physicians' offices or in hospitals before an examination. I find myself exchanging photos of children and grandchildren with perfect strangers and talking about the difficulties in life. Once, while I was setting up an appointment for an exam, I began to chat with the woman who was arranging it for me as she hunched over her computer. I recognized her New York accent, and we began by talking about New York, then the Bush presidency, then her bout with cancer. I hugged her before I left, and when we meet it's like greeting an old friend. When I hold my granddaughter in my arms, I feel a sense of gratitude and of the miraculous. When I observe another person in the fullness of his or her being, regardless of social perceptions, I am also filled with admiration. I marvel not at what he or she may or may not have done but at who that person is, who he or she has become through the tangled web of years and circumstances.

Having time for contemplation has not only enhanced my appreciation of everyday occurrences; it has also helped me become open to new experiences, to see signs of hope and comfort in the most unlikely places. I recently experienced a flare-up and was too tired to feel much of anything, or so I thought. I was preparing a birthday dinner for my husband and unearthed a tablecloth my mother had given us when we were young and that I hadn't used in many years. As I lifted it out of the closet and unfolded it, I admired the handwork, white embroidery on cotton so fine it was almost transparent.

After setting the table, I began the most mundane act of peeling potatoes when suddenly I felt my mother's loving presence, her warmth enfolding me in such a palpable way that it overwhelmed me. It persisted, so I went into my study to meditate and keep that presence a little longer. As I meditated, I realized that I was feeling abandoned in this trying period, but this experience made me wonder how I could have possibly believed that when I had, and continue to have, the profound love of my long-dead mother.

That experience has taught me to remember all the wonderful people who have touched me in this life, as family, as mentors, or as people who have simply showed me kindness. I carry them around, and they too are a source of strength and a reminder that although my condition often seems isolating, I am not alone.

Before I became ill I had a number of close colleagues and friends, but I discovered that it is only in difficult times that we discover our real friends. Not surprisingly, those who stayed with me and who accompany me are the ones who have suffered tragedies themselves. Once, when I was going through a rough period, my friend Ana dropped off a poem she had written about the Cuba she left behind when she had to flee for her life. It was written on handmade paper and embellished with roses her artist brother painted. She also gave me a handmade bookmark with the word "tranquility" embroidered on it and a small book with Renaissance paintings of angels and poetry. She once sent me an article on fibromyalgia with a simple note attached: "You are very brave."

Although I was politically active before my illness, I now understand how significant small gestures can be, a hug or a letter expressing sympathy, and that to accompany a person through a difficult period is to gain a wider life. I can write letters to the children I sponsor through private foreign aid, can spend time mentoring and supporting young people who need help. A telephone call and letters can be just as powerful as attending a rally or gathering signatures. My mother's lesson that we are here for each other has taken on a new resonance. I remember how our house was always filled with people who needed a place to stay and how my mother was always sharing the little we had. That memory and my condition helped me realize that our destinies are not at all separate and that every gesture throbs inside a web that we are part of, regardless of our physical condition.

I now feel that connection in my very being, my whole body. I remember walking down Kedsie Street in Chicago when I was a senior in high school. I was on my way to my mother's office to help her with the invoices when I saw an older man stumble and fall in a doorway across the street. I watched, rooted to the sidewalk, wanting so much to help, but fear overcame me and I walked by. That moment has haunted me all these years. But now I have lost that fear, lost my suppositions about frailty, and see myself reflected in faces that stream by.

One of the greatest changes in values I have experienced has been in my views of success. In the academic world, as in most settings, there is a great emphasis on status and public recognition and an atmosphere of competition that results from such values. Although I was never caught up in those goals, I now feel even more intensely that they are of little consequence to me and keep my distance from such pressures, for I find them very stressful and also distracting. I have gained great respect for the process of work and for the joys of working on collaborative projects. I know that jobs come to an end, acclaim fades, personnel changes occur randomly, and even the best books go out of print. What remains are enduring and invisible acts of kindness. What matters to me now are not social views of success—although every writer needs feedback, needs to know that his or her work has touched others—but wisdom, resilience, and endurance. I know that while I always have a choice of how to respond to situations, I have little control over my body. Thus I feel I have gained understanding and forbearance in this journey, qualities that will serve me in the most demanding situations.

Reinventing myself continually, as I have had to do, has helped me become spiritually powerful and willing to take more risks. Recently my husband and I went to see an exhibit of Claude Monet's later works, experimental paintings he never showed publicly, because of their daring nature, but which he completed from age sixty-five to his eighties. Studying these paintings was like looking at my inner life and at my daily efforts to use my pain as a flying carpet. Instead of the peace and repose of his famous canvases, I was greeted with feverish brushstrokes and wild colors, the oranges, deep blues, and reds anticipating the Fauve movement. Even his proportions had changed; I saw a section of a giant tree trunk cut off by the edges of a massive canvas as if it were growing to eternity. One of the paintings that moved me the most was that of a weeping willow he had completed during World War I. Instead of the usual calm and beautiful proportions of his early work, I saw a raw anguish. Not only the trees were writhing; the whole atmosphere vibrated with ululations.

The very last painting in the exhibit, a giant, wall-length canvas, was just color and depth, as if Monet were tapping solar winds, sunsets, sunrises as he layered oranges and purples of varying profundities. I could see the process: he rendered the scene, then dropped it and just created the feeling of the scene, moving farther and farther away from externals into a deeper reality.

When he completed this work, he was grieving over his wife's death and suffering a debilitating old age and loneliness. Yet in these canvases everything is risk, opening and pushing at limits. It was the unfinished quality, the searching, that pulled at me. Monet's moving reinvention of himself made me realize that without the continual shattering of the known there can be no creation, no true beauty.

❧❧❧

Ironically, while I grieved for many years over what I saw at the time as the loss of my career, it was, in effect, the loss of a way of life and not an ending. I now see my working situation as a blessing. I feel as if I have let go of all my assumed identities and entered my own true self. I don't ever give a thought to my position in society, and as a result experience a wonderful freedom. I think of myself as in the process of becoming and also as belonging to myself, no longer in thrall to social expectations.

One very warm fall, our son gave us frequent-flyer tickets to Hawaii as an anniversary present, and we rented a small apartment on Maui. Our favorite spot was a lava flow called Makina Point at the southernmost tip of the island, which is also a nature reserve. We walked along the coral stones until we reached a cliff and a small shelter of trees. The light seemed to be emanating from the water, and even though the waves were fierce and the coral was sharp and slippery with algae, I felt a yearning to enter that lushness. I didn't have a bathing suit or towel, and in a spurt of joy I peeled off my jeans, T-shirt, tennis shoes, and underwear and stepped into that water. It felt wonderfully alive against my skin, and I reveled in my nakedness. As painful as it has been over the years to strip off every aspect of my social status, it was with utter delight that I returned to a different kind of nakedness. I don't think I would have dared act with such spontaneity in my former life.

Healing is a form of letting go. I don't know how or when I stopped fighting this illness. I only know that there came a time when managing the physical resources I have took center stage while anger and grief moved to the sidelines. Surrender does not mean giving up, but releasing what impedes us in trying to live as well as possible. For me, it means letting go of what I cannot have, not wishing I could live with physical ease as I once did but taking what comes, when it comes, for what it is—a difficult passage, perhaps, or a gift of friendship or inspiration when I least expect it.

The word *surrender* has a negative connotation for many people, but for me it means accepting my situation. When we acknowledge our sorrow, it does not swallow up all our vision and emotion. On the contrary, to experience the complexity of our reality means in essence to transcend it.

Somehow it also means experiencing the grace of recapturing my self-esteem and realizing that I am whole despite my illness, whole in heart and spirit. Whether others see me as such is of lesser importance, for in the solitude that illness imposes one has plenty of time for self-evaluation.

For me, surrendering includes the inexplicable waves of joy I experience periodically for what seems like no reason at all. I may have had a difficult and seemingly empty day and yet I am somehow floating at the end of it, feeling very buoyant inside. I remember telling my husband after returning home from Brandeis and a panel I had organized, "How can I be so happy when I feel so terrible?"

꒲꒲꒲

One summer while in Trieste, my cousins and I visited the Friulian towns of Venzone and Gemona, near the Austrian border. What began as an expedition to see how towns had been reduced to rubble by terrible earthquakes radiating from an epicenter in the Julian Alps turned into a personal pilgrimage for me. As my cousins and I walked through the quiet and orderly streets of Venzone, the mountains rising above seemed benevolent rather than threatening. Only the numbers painted on each stone around the houses and stores gave evidence of the terrible tragedy. They also revealed the skilled efforts of restoration that were still taking place since the catastrophe that occurred in July 1976. Everything that remained intact was painstakingly removed from the debris and catalogued for future use, so that the town and its beautiful cathedral are now a combination of the ancient and new.

As we entered the Duomo of San Andrea Apostolo on the central piazza of Venzone, I saw a new ceiling on the central nave but also walls with swaths of masonry like patches over huge wounds, and frescoes that were still in tatters. It was as if I were seeing torn flesh. As I stood beside the altar, the mountain loomed through windows whose stained glass had not yet been replaced, destruction and creation intertwined in a way that shook me by the roots. This was not the home of a crucified Christ but a crucified population, so many of whom had died beneath the rubble.

On the side of the altar a sculptor had taken a single 150-year old cedar felled by lightning and transformed it into a group of men, women, and children huddled in a circle with arms raised to the heavens in supplication. It was intended to represent the population of Venzone begging the Creator to spare them another earthquake, but to me it was a war memorial as well as an homage to suffering humanity. The circle of tormented and huge outstretched hands resonated inside me. I felt I was witnessing my own journey and that of so many others who have had to rebuild their lives as refugees, as survivors of wars, of illnesses, of the tragedies that rain down indiscriminately on so many of us. The unfinished church was more beautiful because it was not paradise I was seeking but reality, a facet of it that is so often deliberately hidden.

The nearby town of Gemona was also destroyed, "All in One Night," as the newspaper article and photos revealed on a panel inside the Duomo Santa Maria Assunta, a thirteenth-century church. It was hard to believe from the crushed stones visible in this photo a town could have been re-constructed, but as we strolled through the streets, they were humming with activity. The pillars of the church were left standing, though tilted, and the church was painstakingly rebuilt on them. The mountain of San Simeone loomed threateningly above the church. It too seemed tilted and apparently had lost twenty meters of height. However, the surviving pop-ulation chose to stay despite the risks of yet another earthquake.

Astonishingly, many of the sculptured figures on the front of the cathe-dral were partly preserved, including two stone monks from the twelfth century on either side of the stairs leading to the church door. Dressed in their rough, worn habits and capes, they spoke to me of dignity and sur-vival. Inside the church, the slanted pillars and a hanging Christ were searing reminders of the human condition. The cross was missing, and the figure of Christ was without forearms and had lost its legs below the knees, a broken body suspended behind a glass wall as a testimony to our suffering. I found it beautiful.

So many people turn away in fear from those in wheelchairs or strug-gling with walkers, or who have difficulty controlling their facial expres-sions. I have learned to look for the inner core of each person and find faces and bodies without masks more beautiful than supposedly flawless ones. My son's friend Brad, who has a severe case of multiple sclerosis, worries continually about his appearance, but I find that he has become more handsome than ever since his illness and that his face has deepened. My husband took photos of him and his family while on a visit, and we were struck by the strength in his expression. To look with understand-ing at a person like Brad is to see our own depths, the secret self we hide beneath a constructed exterior.

That is how much I have changed: I see meaning in circumstances others might find frightening, see myself in the process of transformation, see a continuity beyond my own small episode on this earth. Neither my goal nor the path was laid out, but in the hourly, daily, monthly, yearly process of coping, I began a lonely process of searching. If it often seemed as if I were walking in the dark, this search has nevertheless brought me to a profound realization of the divinity within me and around me, to a reality that is vast and invisible. I have found this insight to be the gift that comes from accepting the terms of our journey.